CW00368872

NEW ADVANCED FIRST-AID

By the same authors

NEW ESSENTIAL FIRST AID (1984). London; Pan

NEW ADVANCED FIRST-AID

A. WARD GARDNER, MD, FRCPI, FFOM, DIH

with

PETER J. ROYLANCE, RD, MB, CHB, FIBIOL,
DIPPHARMMED

Illustrations by
Michael Stokes

THIRD EDITION

WRIGHT
BRISTOL
1984

Published by,
John Wright & Sons Ltd, 823–825 Bath Road,
Bristol BS4 5NU, England.

Second edition, 1977
Third edition, 1984

Gardner, A. Ward
New advanced first-aid.—3rd ed.
1. First aid in illness and injury
I. Title   II. Roylance, Peter J.
616.02′52   RC87

British Library Cataloguing in Publication Data

ISBN 0 7236 0803 2

Library of Congress Catalog Card Number: 84-50391

Printed in Great Britain by
Henry Ling Limited
at The Dorset Press, Dorchester

PREFACE

*It is a great advantage for a system of
philosophy to be substantially true.*
GEORGE SANTAYANA

This book is designed as a companion to *New Essential First
Aid*. The aim is to provide information about first-aid in
greater depth and over a wider field. We assume that the
reader has a good grasp of *essential* first-aid and has read and
understood the basic information which is given in *New
Essential First Aid*.

As well as widening the scope of the subjects covered, we
have tried to give some of the reasons why things should
be done in this or that way, and more explanations of the
underlying principles. We have included first-aid procedures additional to those carried out by trained first-aiders
which, under normal circumstances, would be carried out
only by trained nurses or doctors. But first-aid is for nurses
and doctors too!

For the expert first-aider, a knowledge of these procedures
will be useful background information. For example, giving
intravenous fluids, including saline, plasma and blood,
could be a part of first-aid—but will normally be done only
by a doctor or under his immediate direction. The advanced
first-aider should, however, be aware of the circumstances
when such procedures can be employed with advantage. An
advanced first-aider could be a nurse or a doctor who, away
from full medical facilities, may have to give first-aid. We

have also assumed that any first-aid will be carried out in a place from where skilled medical help is but a few hours away. This book is *not* intended to give instruction in what to do if medical help is unobtainable—for example, in lonely parts of the world or at sea. For such circumstances quite a different sort of book is required.

There are in the text a number of deliberate omissions. These include:

lifting and handling—this can best be learned in practical training sessions;

nursing procedures—because they are not normally within the scope of first aid; and

the technique of stomach washouts—because we believe that this should only be done by experienced and highly trained medical or nursing staff.

The use by first-aiders of Guedel-type airways has been relegated to an appendix because, after much discussion, our anaesthetist colleagues have persuaded us that their dangers in semi-skilled hands can outweigh their advantages. Unless special *practical* instruction is given in the use of these airways, we prefer to omit their use.

First-aid is a subject which has to be read, understood, thought about and practised *before* emergencies arise. The difference between the expert and the uninitiated—in first-aid, as in other fields—lies in the capacity of the expert to analyse any situation so that he can fit his responses smoothly and with a minimum of hurry and apparent effort to the varying situations which confront him, and to organize the responses of others in a way which will benefit the situation, in addition to just knowing what to do.

We hope that this book may help to generate expertise, and that it is, and will remain, useful to those wishing to learn more and keep up to date in first-aid. We would therefore welcome ideas, comments and criticisms, and would be most grateful to be told of possible improvements. If you like this book, or if you do not like it, or if you have any views or ideas and would like to tell us, please write to us at

John Wright & Sons Ltd,
The Stonebridge Press,
823–825 Bath Road,
Bristol BS4 5NU.

A. WARD GARDNER
PETER J. ROYLANCE

Acknowledgements

We wish to thank all the people who have helped in preparing this book, and are especially grateful to:
The late Dr J. Apley, CBE; Mr Jason G. Brice, FRCS; Professor G. V. P. Chamberlain, FRCS, MRCOG; Dr K. J. Collins; Dr J. L. J: de Bary; Mr L. W. Downer; Dr A. Downie; Dr K. C. Easton, OBE; Dr E. F. Edson; Professor A. P. M. Forrest; the late Mr F. R. Frewin; Miss Mary D. Gardner, BSc, FRIC; Surgeon Captain E. C. Glover, VRD, FRCS, DOMS; Mr Kenneth G. Jamieson, MS, FRACS; Dr J. G. Jesson; Dr Eric Jones-Evans; Mr L. G. Lewis; Dr J. W. Lloyd; Dr O. J. S. Macdonald; Mr E. A. Malkin, FRCS, DLO; Dr T. M. Moles; Chief Fire Officer George Nash, Grad I Fire E; the late Dr H. Alistair Reid, OBE; Dr John Tonge; Dr Joan Whelan; Mrs E. Williams, and the Editor, *The Journal of the Society of Occupational Medicine*.

CONTENTS

CHAPTER 1

RESUSCITATION

For I perceive the way to life lies here;
Come, pluck up, Heart; let's neither faint
nor fear :
Better, tho' difficult, th' right way to go,
Then wrong, though easie, when the end
is wo'.
JOHN BUNYAN

INTRODUCTION

When any casualty becomes unconscious, cannot breathe or his heart stops beating, he is in need of urgent first-aid.

These three conditions may come on together very suddenly as a result of electrocution, or more slowly and one at a time due to entering an atmosphere in which there is insufficient oxygen.

The rate of return to normal function or consciousness may be swift or slow depending on circumstances. In every case, however, there will be a gap in normal functioning which should be bridged by the appropriate first-aid measures. These measures may include resuscitation.

The term resuscitation includes the giving of oxygen, intravenous fluids ('drips'), blood transfusions, artificial respiration, heart compression and other medical procedures. All resuscitation procedures have this in common: they are required suddenly in an emergency and must be swiftly and correctly carried out in order to be life-saving.

It is essential, therefore, that you know exactly what to do and that you have practised doing it before the emergency arises. It is unlikely that you will succeed in resuscitation unless you do the right things in the right order, and do them swiftly and correctly.

1

THE THREE BRIDGES OF FIRST-AID

Any casualty who is unable to

—keep his airway clear of obstruction (move or cough)

or

—circulate his blood (heart beating)

or

—shift air in and out of his lungs (breathe)

will probably die unless the appropriate first-aid procedure which can bridge the gap in normal functions is carried out, or unless perchance the condition rapidly corrects itself.

Table 1.1 shows the casualty's need, the reason for his failure to meet the need, and the remedy in first-aid to bridge the gap in normal functioning.

TABLE 1.1

Casualty's need	Reason for failure to fulfil need	First-aid treatment
To keep his airway clear of obstruction—to be able to cough, move, swallow and spit	Unconsciousness from any cause	*first bridge* Place casualty in the unconscious position, clear the mouth of dentures, debris, loose natural teeth, blood or vomit and apply a slight head-down tip
To circulate blood—to have the heart beating	Electrocution, heart attack, deep un-consciousness from any cause	*second bridge* Heart compression
To shift air in and out of the lungs—to breathe	Deep unconscious-ness, obstructed breathing, electrocu-tion, drowning and so on	*third bridge* Artificial respiration by the mouth-to-nose or mouth-to-mouth method

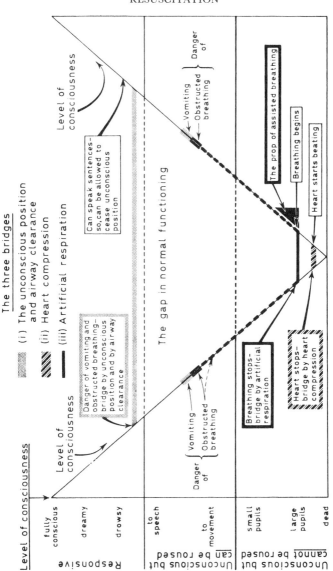

Figure 1.1.—The three bridges

Figure 1.1 shows the three bridges across the gap.

The first bridge, THE UNCONSCIOUS POSITION, must be used, if possible, in anticipation of vomiting and obstructed breathing. If the casualty is found to be breathing but unconscious, he should at once be placed in the unconscious position with a slight head-down tip, *and* with full neck extension, and the airway should be cleared (*Figure 1.2*). In this position any secretions, blood or vomit will tend

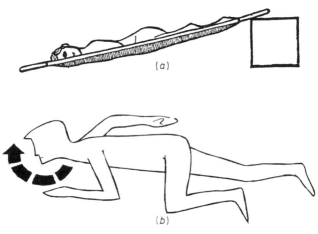

Figure 1.2.—The unconscious position. (a) Apply a head-down tip. (b) Full head and neck extension in teeth-clenched position to keep airway clear

to flow out of the mouth or nose and will neither obstruct the airway nor pool in the back of the throat, whence it could syphon into the air passages and lungs. The unconscious position thus maintains a clear airway, and is the position into which all unconscious casualties must be turned. The casualty should be kept in this position until he regains near full consciousness, as measured by his ability to speak sentences. For the treatment of vomiting in an unconscious casualty, *see* page 17.

VOMITING FOLLOWING RECOVERY FROM DEEP UNCON-SCIOUSNESS

Because the vomiting centre in the brain, having been inactive during deep unconsciousness, becomes revitalized during recovery, vomiting may occur at this time. Airway obstruction due to vomiting is thus a constant threat to life in the recovery period. Prevent airway obstruction by the use of the unconscious position with a head-down tip. If vomiting has occurred, treat it as outlined on page 17.

a word about priorities

> Heart compression and
> artificial respiration are
> **TOP PRIORITY**
> first-aid procedures

Failure to do heart compression and artificial respiration *at once* on any casualty whose heart is not beating or failure to do artificial respiration *at once* on any casualty who is not breathing may easily result in loss of life. Delay, often needless, is among the commonest causes of failures of these procedures.

The second bridge, HEART COMPRESSION, is used when the heart stops beating. The heart may suddenly stop beating, for example, following a heart attack or following electro-cution.

HEART COMPRESSION

The AIM of HEART COMPRESSION is to do the work of the heart in a casualty whose heart has stopped beating.

Heart compression is effected by squeezing the heart between the breastbone at the front and the spine at the back. With each compression, blood is squeezed out of the heart and round the body.

In order to carry out heart compression it is necessary to—

(1) Act *immediately*.

(2) Check that the heart has stopped beating.

(3) Carry out artificial respiration in addition to heart compression. (*See* below.)

(4) Place the casualty lying on his back on a hard surface.

(5) When the chest is falling after each inflation apply six rapid pressures to the lower half of the breastbone.

(6) Continue to apply heart compression after each inflation until the heart starts to beat.

(7) Continue artificial respiration until breathing starts.

(8) Turn the casualty, when breathing, into the unconscious position.

(9) Watch carefully to see that the heart does not stop again and that breathing continues.

(10) Arrange for the casualty to be taken to hospital, still watching carefully to see that heart beat and breathing are maintained.

(1) *Act immediately*

When the heart stops, 2–4 minutes at the most is the likely balance time between life and death, unless effective action is taken. It follows, therefore, that there must be *no delay* in applying heart compression when the heart stops beating.

(2) *Check that the heart has stopped beating*

Quickly check that the following signs are present before doing heart compression.

6

(i) The casualty is unconscious.

(ii) Heart sounds cannot be heard and no pulse can be felt. You have to practise these things *before* an emergency arises. Listen over the left side of the chest for heart sounds. The sounds are rather low and rumbling and have been likened in rhythm to the sounds 'lub-dup'. Try to listen for heart sounds in a few of your friends so that you know what to listen for! Absence of these sounds means that the heart is not beating. Any *regular* sound in the chest is probably a heart sound. Practise also feeling the pulse.

(iii) Breathing has stopped, or only feeble gasps are made.

(iv) The pupils are large (dilated).

If you think that the heart has stopped suddenly, no pulse can be felt, and the casualty gasps or stops breathing and looks dead, *do not wait for the pupils to dilate but get on at once with giving heart compression and artificial respiration.*

It is much better, in any case where you think that the heart may be stopped, to get on *at once* with the job of resuscitation without waiting for the pupils to dilate. A death-like appearance with absent pulse and absent or gasping breathing should always be treated as an indication for *immediate action* to give heart compression and artificial respiration. Gasping breathing may go on for a very short time after the heart has stopped suddenly.

The best rule is, if
    —the casualty is unconscious,
    —no pulse can be felt, or heart sounds heard,
    —breathing has stopped, or is only in gasps
DO NOT WASTE TIME by further checking
START HEART COMPRESSION AT ONCE—
if in doubt do it; he may die if you do not.

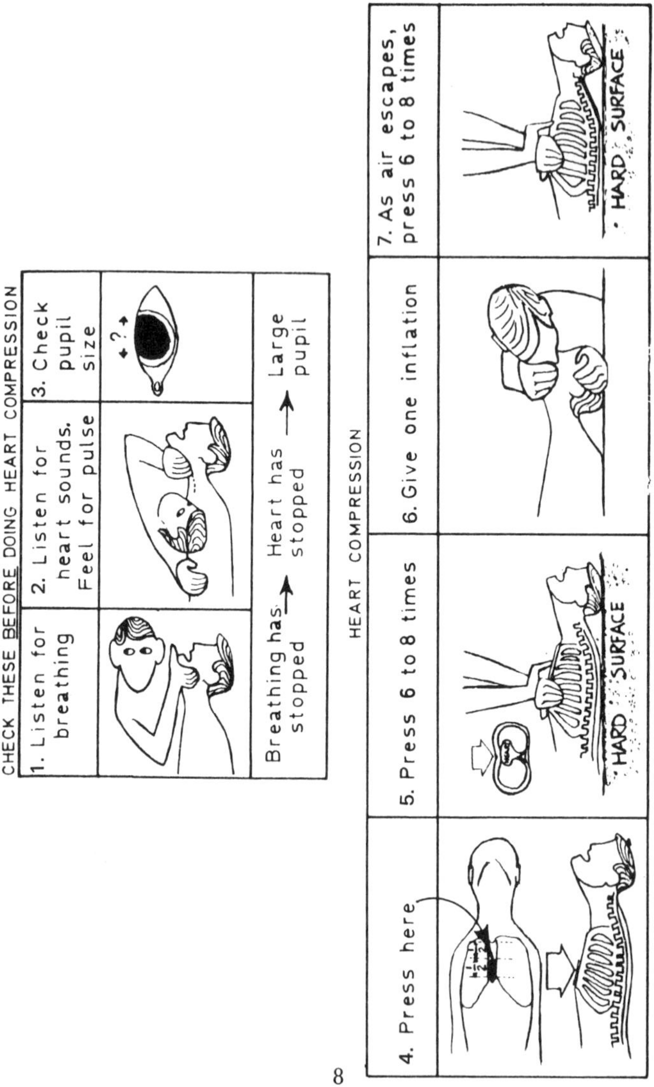

CHECK THESE BEFORE DOING HEART COMPRESSION

1. Listen for breathing	2. Listen for heart sounds. Feel for pulse	3. Check pupil size

Breathing has stopped → Heart has stopped → Large pupil

HEART COMPRESSION

4. Press here	5. Press 6 to 8 times	6. Give one inflation	7. As air escapes, press 6 to 8 times

Figure 1.3.–*Heart compression*

8

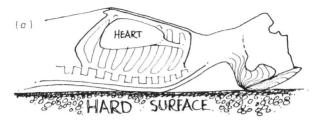

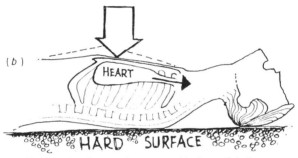

Figure 1.4.—Compression squeezes blood out of the heart

(3) *Carry out artificial respiration in addition to heart compression*

If the heart has stopped, breathing will also have stopped. *Heart compression should never be given alone; artificial respiration must always be given as well.*

(4) *Place the casualty lying on his back on a hard surface*

Blood must be squeezed out of the heart by compressing the heart between the breastbone in front and the spine behind *(Figure 1.4)*. Therefore, if pressure is to be effective, the casualty must be lying on a non-yielding hard surface, for example, a floor or table. A very soft springy bed will not do—the casualty is simply pushed into the soft bed and no compression will occur.

9

(5) *When the chest is falling after each inflation, apply six rapid pressures to the lower half of the breastbone*

First, find the top of the breastbone by locating the notch. Next, find the lower end from where the ribs spread out. Ignore the little 'tail' of the breastbone. Now measure off the lower half of the breastbone and place the heel of one hand on the breastbone at the mid-point of the lower half. Place the heel of the other hand on top of the hand which is on the breastbone. Now, *but only in emergency, never in practice,* press 6–8 times, each sufficient in an adult to produce an inward (downward) movement of the lower part of the breastbone of about 4 cm ($1\frac{1}{2}$ inches). The pressures should be about 2 per second in an adult. Allowing for stops to inflate the lungs, this should produce a heart rate of about 90 per minute. It is better to aim for a high rather than a low heart rate.

Children will require faster rates than adults—say, about 3 pressures per second, to give a heart rate of about 120 per minute.

If you are exerting the correct short, sharp downward pressure, the casualty will tend to make a grunting sound with each downward pressure, as air will also be forced out of the chest.

CAUTION

Never practise the pressing part of this procedure on conscious people. You may do serious damage. Casualties who are not breathing and whose hearts have stopped are relaxed to a degree which permits such movement without damage. A conscious person is not relaxed, and pressing should not therefore be attempted.

When pressing, aim to produce a sudden sharp downward pressure of the correct amount, which is suddenly released. A representation of the type of pressure required is

The downward pressures are short and sharp. Slow ups and downs like a wave

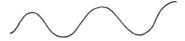

will not move blood from the heart nearly as well as short sharp pressures. The downward strokes should be rather like those used in pumping up a tyre with a bicycle pump—quick, sharp and released suddenly.

Practise finding the lower half of the breastbone and laying on the hands correctly. But NEVER press, except on an unconscious casualty whose heart has stopped—that is, in a real emergency.

In the case of children, light one-handed pressure only should be applied. Babies require only thumb pressure. Use the fleshy part of the thumb, not the hard tip. The methods for doing heart compression in children and babies are given on pages 13 and 14.

Always be gentle. Never use more force than is required to produce a movement of the breastbone sufficient to compress the heart—in an adult about $2\frac{1}{2}$–4 cm (1–$1\frac{1}{2}$ inches).

(6) *Continue to apply heart compression after each inflation until the heart starts to beat*

Early signs of success in the application of heart compression are

—the pupils get smaller, and

—the colour of the casualty improves. A change in colour from blueness or greyness towards pinkness is an improvement.

In order to find out if the heart has started to beat, it is necessary to make a brief stop in carrying out heart compression. Such stops should be very short and no longer than is required to find out if the heart is beating. You must know how to check heart beat, and must practise doing this *before* an emergency arises. Listen with your ear against the left side of the chest for heart sounds and feel for a pulse beat in the arteries of the neck, elbow or wrist. Any one of these may give the necessary information, but one may be easier to carry out in any particular case. All should be practised.

If the heart is beating, stop heart compression.

pupil size as a guide to brain oxygenation

The pupils dilate (enlarge) within about 45 seconds of oxygen cut-off to the brain. In a similar way, the pupils will constrict (grow smaller) within about 45 seconds of *adequate* oxygen reaching the brain, that is when circulation and breathing are restored—if necessary by carrying out heart compression and artificial respiration.

Failure of the pupils to constrict is a sign that circulation of oxygen-containing blood to the brain is ineffective. A change in size towards smaller pupils will indicate success.

(7) Continue artificial respiration until breathing starts

Place your ear near the casualty's nose or mouth and listen to check for breathing. At the same time, a glance along the top of the chest is probably the best method to detect movement. Watch particularly the upper abdomen, just below where the ribs separate. A very small downward movement of the diaphragm, as in weak breathing, will produce a rise in this part of the abdomen even when there is very little or no apparent chest movement.

(8) Turn the casualty, when breathing, into the unconscious position

When you are sure that the casualty needs no further artificial respiration—nor small puffs to assist weak breathing —turn him into the unconscious position with a slight head-down tip if possible. Make sure that the head is fully back and the chin is raised in the teeth clenched position to keep the air passages free of obstruction. This follows the general rules for the treatment of unconsciousness.

(9) *Watch carefully to see that the heart does not stop again and that breathing continues*

After the heart has stopped beating and has restarted, it may easily stop again. Similarly, breathing can easily stop again. You must watch the casualty very carefully and be prepared to restart heart compression or artificial respiration, or both, at a moment's notice.

(10) *Arrange for the casualty to be taken to hospital, still watching carefully to see that heart beat and breathing are maintained*

Do not be in too much of a hurry to move the casualty until you are *sure* that breathing and heart beat are reasonably established. On the other hand, do not delay sending the casualty to hospital for any longer than is absolutely necessary. Check regularly to make sure that the heart continues to beat. Careful observations and readiness to restart heart compression and artificial respiration will be required until the casualty arrives safely in hospital.

HEART COMPRESSION IN CHILDREN AND BABIES

Compressing the heart by pressure on the lower half of the breastbone is carried out in children and babies by different methods from those used in the adult because much less force is required. One hand only should be used for pressing on children. The force used should be light and should aim to produce a smaller movement than in the adult. In babies, thumb or finger pressure only should be used.

a note about the importance of speed in starting heart compression

To be successful, heart compression must be started IMMEDIATELY the heart stops beating. Conversely, lack

13

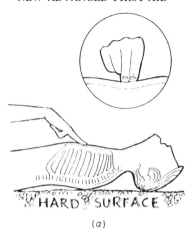

HARD SURFACE

(a)

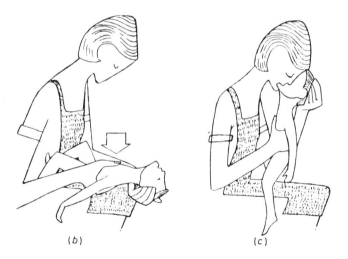

(b)   (c)

Figure 1.5.—(a) For children, use two fingers only. (b) For infants, use thumb pressure only. (c) Cover both nose and mouth when inflating

14

of success is due to DELAY in applying heart compression. Doctors who have studied this problem believe that

> *the commonest avoidable cause of failure*
> —and perhaps worse, of vegetable survival of the body when the brain is dead—
> *is NEEDLESS delay in applying heart compression.*

It is therefore worth repeating that any casualties who are *not breathing* should be given artificial respiration at once. If the cause of not breathing is *electrocution*, or if the *colour does not improve after a few inflations*, the casualty should be checked to establish whether the heart is beating or not.

If *no pulse is felt* and *no heart sounds* can be heard, and the *pupils are widely dilated*, there must be

NO DELAY
in starting HEART COMPRESSION

The time which separates life from death under these conditions *may* be as long as 2 minutes—but may also be *much less*. Every second counts; start heart compression in addition to artificial respiration at the earliest possible moment. Your reward may be to save a life.

capillary refilling after lip compression

When the red margin of the lip is compressed by a finger pressing the lip against the teeth, a white patch will be seen when the finger is removed. This white patch will in a normal person, be seen to fill immediately with red from the edges inwards, until the lip resumes normal colour. Witness the phenomenon in yourself—press the lower lip firmly for about one second and then watch in a mirror the refilling of the small (capillary) blood vessels which occurs as soon as the pressure is released.

Capillary refilling after lip compression depends on an adequate circulation of blood—and hence on heartbeat. Slow, inadequate or absent capillary refilling will therefore be due to inadequate heart beat in the absence of some obvious local cause of blanching, such as extreme cold or injury to the part.

This is a quick and easy test to perform, and should be more generally used as a test of circulation. A similar phenomenon can be seen in the nail beds by pinching the fingers or toes—but is more difficult to reproduce and observe in a reliable way.

The third bridge, *ARTIFICIAL RESPIRATION*, should always be used if a casualty is not breathing. As soon as the casualty begins to breathe weakly, the prop of assisted breathing should be used until he can breathe strongly and quite independently.

Assisted breathing is the technique of giving artificial respiration *in time with* the casualty's own weak breathing attempts.

The fact that any casualty is *not breathing* must be recognized at once. There must then be no delay in applying artificial respiration by the mouth-to-nose or mouth-to-mouth methods.

If the casualty's colour does not improve after about six inflations, find out if the heart is beating (*see* pages 6 and 7). If the heart is not beating, *heart compression* must be carried out in addition to artificial respiration (*see* pages 8 and 9).

VOMITING AS A COMPLICATION OF ARTIFICIAL RESPIRATION

Vomiting may occur before or during artificial respiration. There is some evidence that regurgitant vomiting due to stomach inflation is less frequent following mouth-to-nose inflation. We therefore recommend the mouth-to-nose method as the first choice both because it is easier to do and in the hope of preventing this complication.

TREATING AN UNCONSCIOUS CASUALTY WHO HAS VOMITED

If vomiting occurs or has occurred, the first need is to clear the airway.

—*Turn the casualty into the unconscious position* with full neck extension and a head-down tip if possible.

—*Clear the airway.* Remove dentures if present and, if possible, *use a sucker* to get rid of vomit (*see* page 23). If a sucker is not available, mop out the vomit, using a handkerchief or any other soft cloth. If nothing else is available, use your fingers.

—*Inflate the lungs* as soon as the airway is thought to be clear enough, if the casualty does not breathe as soon as the airway is thought to be clear. Artificial respiration can be given in the unconscious position or with the casualty lying on his back.

—*Continue to suck or mop out the airway to try to keep it clear.* If the airway can be kept clear, the casualty may then be turned onto his back if more convenient.

If you think that vomiting may occur, it may be wise to give artificial respiration to such a casualty in the unconscious position. In this way, obstructed breathing is less likely to occur.

A note about tubes and airways for use in artificial respiration

There is no doubt that certain apparatus can be used in carrying out mouth-to-nose or mouth-to-mouth artificial respiration, and that this apparatus helps to secure an adequate airway and serves to overcome some of the aesthetic objections to the method. However, people who have been trained to carry out mouth-to-mouth artificial respiration using a tube or airway may waste valuable seconds looking for these, instead of getting on *at*

17

once with doing the artificial respiration. On occasions, people have even failed to carry out artificial respiration when no tube was available.

For these reasons, and also because very adequate ventilation can be obtained without any apparatus, we prefer—as a first-aid procedure—to teach artificial respiration *without* the use of tubes and airways. We have, however, included some remarks in appendix 1 for those who may wish to use apparatus.

Giving artificial respiration to a casualty who has had a tracheotomy

Very occasionally, a casualty may be encountered who breathes through a hole in the front of the neck situated at about the collar-stud level. This hole is the result of an operation called a tracheotomy. Such casualties should be given artificial respiration by breathing into the hole in the neck, because this is the way that air gets in and out of their lungs. There is usually no need to cover the mouth or close off the nose of such casualties, unless air is heard escaping by these routes. Apart from blowing into the hole in the neck, the technique of artificial respiration is similar to that normally used. Extra care should be taken to see that the hole in the neck does not become blocked, especially when turning the casualty into the unconscious position.

CIRCULATORY STAGNATION

MEDICAL INFORMATION

Stagnation of blood can arise in two main ways.

Following stoppage of heart beat

This results in *generalized* stagnation.

As a result of trapping or crushing injuries

This results in *localized* stagnation. When the trapping or crushing is relieved, stagnant blood—perhaps in large amounts—may be released into the general circulating blood.

18

STAGNANT BLOOD IS OXYGEN-DEFICIENT ACID BLOOD

The basic cause of the rise in acidity of stagnant blood is lack of oxygen in the blood and tissues. Available supplies are soon used up if blood does not circulate.

Two main processes are involved.

Carbon dioxide continues to be produced in the tissues, but is not taken away by the stagnant blood. This gas in solution in blood—as *carbonic acid*—causes a rise in acidity.

Other products of tissue activity in an oxygen-deficient or oxygen-lacking medium give rise to substances which are acid. Until oxygen-rich circulating blood is restored, the acidity of the blood will be raised.

The *volume* of stagnant blood and the duration of *stagnation* will together determine the rise in acidity. If an appreciable rise in acidity of the blood occurs following the release of stagnant blood into the circulating blood a serious condition (*metabolic acidosis*) is present.

We can therefore say in summary that stagnant blood is deficient in oxygen and is more acid when compared with normal blood.

One effect of 'acid blood' is to affect heart beat. Heart beat may be impaired, or may actually stop, because of raised blood acidity. *'Acid blood' can thus precipitate or perpetuate stoppage of heart beat.*

The treatment of circulatory stagnation falls into three sections.

Restore the circulation.

Restore oxygen to the blood and tissues.

Reduce the acidity of the blood.

Restore the circulation

General stagnation.—This will be due to stoppage of heart beat and should be treated by heart compression (page 8).

19

Local stagnation.—This will be due to crushing or trapping, and the treatment will be to remove the cause of the crushing. General problems of metabolic acidosis will only arise following crush injury to large areas or following crushing of moderate areas which have been trapped for some time—say, an hour or longer.

Restore oxygen to the blood and tissues

After circulation has been restored, the amount of oxygen in the blood and tissues depends on

the efficiency of breathing, and

the concentration of oxygen breathed in.

—the efficiency of breathing

All the measures which relieve obstructed breathing and which help breathing—posture, for example—may be of importance, because oxygen must first be breathed in before it can be absorbed into the blood and circulated to the tissues (page 22).

—the concentration of oxygen breathed in

The oxygen concentration of about 20 per cent in air is normally adequate to keep the blood and the tissues fully supplied with oxygen. However, following the accumulation of a *severe oxygen debt*, such as will arise due to circulatory stagnation following other than momentary stoppage of heart beat or following severe crush injury, oxygen in higher concentrations should be given in an attempt to restore oxygen to the blood and tissues as quickly as possible. Other conditions which may give rise to severe oxygen debt—and thus to metabolic acidosis—are chest injuries and brain injuries. The mechanism in these cases is that normal breathing is greatly impaired. The giving of oxygen in first-aid is discussed on page 21.

Reduce the acidity of the blood

The acidity of the blood can be reduced by injecting a solution of sodium bicarbonate. As soon as circulation has been restored and the casualty is breathing, an intravenous injection of 100 ml of 8·4 per cent *wt/vol* (molar) sodium bicarbonate solution* should be given if a doctor is available and this is possible.

Further injections of 100 ml of the same solution may be required if heart beat tends to fail again, if the amount of stagnant blood is large, if the duration of stagnation is long, or if the circulation again becomes poor or stagnant. Not more than 300 ml should be given.

A note should always be sent to the hospital stating the amount of sodium bicarbonate solution which has been given.

THE USE OF OXYGEN IN FIRST AID

Air contains about 20 per cent of oxygen. This concentration of oxygen is adequate under normal circumstances, and in most abnormal circumstances, to sustain life. But, for the oxygen in air to be used effectively by the body, the air passages must be free and unobstructed and the air must be breathed in and out of the lungs in adequate quantities.

The effectiveness of the 20 per cent of oxygen which is in air should not be overlooked by those who happen to be in possession of oxygen-giving apparatus. Provided that the airway is clear and unobstructed, and that respiratory movements can take place normally, fresh air will usually supply adequate amounts of oxygen.

There are five common indications for the use of oxygen in first-aid.

   (*i*) Blueness (cyanosis) which is NOT caused by *obstructed breathing* nor by *inadequate or absent breathing movements*.

  (*ii*) Following severe chest injuries, severe head injuries or severe bleeding.

 (*iii*) Following heart attacks or stoppage of circulation.

 (*iv*) Carbon monoxide gassing (coal gas).

   (*v*) Asthma from whatever cause.

---

* This solution is available in 100 ml ampoules. It contains 1 mEq of sodium bicarbonate per ml.

(i) Blueness which is NOT due to airway obstruction or to inadequate or absent breathing movements

In first-aid, LACK OF OXYGEN which results in blueness (cyanosis) is usually due to AIRWAY OB-STRUCTION or to inadequate or absent breathing movements.

These causes of lack of oxygen should be discovered and corrected before any attempt is made to administer oxygen. We would emphasize that blueness of the lips, ear-tips and nail-beds, or indeed blueness of the whole skin, are not reasons for giving oxygen.

Oxygen should not normally be given until after

—air passages are cleared—by removing dentures, debris, foreign bodies and by sucking out or otherwise removing blood, vomit or secretions, and by getting the head fully back with the mouth shut and the teeth clenched to open the airway.

—breathing is assisted as far as possible—by using posture to best advantage to aid breathing, by closing open chest wounds and by fixing unstable segments of the chest wall (pages 101–105).

If, however, in spite of these efforts the casualty's colour does not improve, there is then a need to give artificial respiration and/or oxygen.

The use of a sucker to clear the airway should be a much more widely used and practised procedure (page 106 and *Figure 1.6*).

Remember when looking for blueness that a good light is essential. Mild degrees of blueness may not be recognized under poor lighting conditions even by experienced people. In casualties whose skin is brown or black, blueness may be very difficult to spot, but the colour of the lips and inside of the mouth may show blueness.

Blueness should be looked for especially in any casualty

—who is unconscious

—has a chest injury.

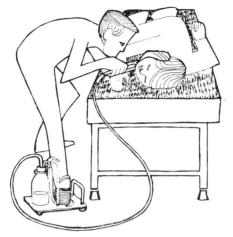

Figure 1.6.—Clear the airway by using a sucker

(*ii*) *Following severe head injuries, severe chest injuries or severe bleeding*

In severe head or chest injuries, or severe bleeding, the amount of oxygen reaching the tissues may be inadequate and giving oxygen may help to raise the amount of oxygen which reaches the tissues.

Casualties who have *serious head and/or chest injuries* are especially liable to suffer from oxygen-lack as a result of inadequate movement of air in and out of the lungs. This oxygen-lack may be remediable by carrying out the procedures described previously, which can remedy obstructed breathing, and can make best use of posture and so on. However, many *serious* head and chest injury casualties will still require all the help that can be given to get oxygen into their tissues, and will thus require oxygen administration, *after* all the aforementioned procedures have been carried out. Casualties who have *bled severely* may also suffer from oxygen-lack in the tissues—which is especially felt in the brain—

23

as a result of deficient oxygen-carrying capacity due to lack of red blood cells. Oxygen may therefore benefit these casualties.

(iii) Following heart attacks or stoppage of circulation

Oxygen, if available, should be given as soon as possible to any casualty who has suffered a severe heart attack (page 177), or whose heart has, or may have, stopped beating, regardless of whether they show any sign of blueness or have a normal or pale colour. Heart compression should, of course, be carried out *at once* on any casualty whose heart has stopped beating, and oxygen should then be given, if available.

Immediately on release from crushing or trapping injuries which involve as much as a whole leg or more, a considerable volume of oxygen-deficient blood may enter the circulation. Giving oxygen during release and immediately afterwards for 5–10 minutes will help to avert any generalized oxygen deficiency which may thus arise.

(iv) Carbon monoxide gassing

Casualties who have been overcome by carbon monoxide should be given oxygen until they reach hospital. It is important to realize that such casualties will suffer from severe oxygen-lack in the tissues. This is because carbon monoxide combines with haemoglobin—the oxygen-carrying part of blood. The haemoglobin which is converted to carboxyhaemoglobin cannot be used for oxygen transport—and the worse the gassing the more carboxyhaemoglobin will be produced. Oxygen hastens the conversion of carboxyhaemoglobin and if the oxygen is given in a compression chamber (hyperbaric oxygen), this may reduce the late effects of lack of oxygen to the brain.

(v) Asthma

Asthma is characterized by wheezy, difficult and distressed breathing. Oxygen may help such casualties when their breathing is very distressed, but before giving oxygen they should be placed in a sitting position as shown on page 104. Worry, excitement and emotional tension often play a large part in the precipitation of asthmatic attacks so attempts should always be made to reassure the casualty and to comfort him.

The indiscriminate use of oxygen in first-aid, especially when it is used as a substitute for an unobstructed airway and proper airway clearance, must be avoided. As with any other procedure, the advanced first-aider must have a clear idea of what he is doing and why. We have therefore summarized the preceding discussion by producing the following

rule for the use of oxygen in first-aid

OXYGEN should be given to casualties with
—BLUENESS which is NOT RELIEVED in the presence of a
    free airway and/or
    adequate breathing movements
and to casualties who have
—SEVERE HEAD and/or CHEST INJURY or have BLED SEVERELY
—HEART ATTACK or STOPPAGE of CIRCULATION
or who have been
—GASSED by CARBON MONOXIDE
or suffered from
—ASTHMA, severely.

Last, if airway obstruction cannot be relieved, oxygen may be tried; however, it is usually more important to try to relieve the airway obstruction than to give oxygen under these circumstances.

It follows from this rule that casualties who suffer from blueness should

> *first*, be checked to see that they are not suffering from obstructed breathing. If they are suffering from obstructed breathing, appropriate treatment should at once be instituted.
>
> *second*, be checked to see that breathing movements are present and adequate; if not, they should be treated by attention to their chest injuries or by artificial respiration or assisted breathing.
>
> *third*, be given oxygen.

a warning note

The normal stimulus to breathing is the amount of carbon dioxide present in the blood. It happens occasionally, however, that a casualty who has had difficulty in breathing—usually for some time—may stop breathing after he has been given oxygen. This is because the stimulus to breathing in this casualty was oxygen-lack.

Artificial respiration should, of course, be given at once to any casualty who has stopped breathing.

A casualty who is not blue, and who has neither suffered a heart attack nor stoppage of heart beat, and who has not been gassed by carbon monoxide nor suffers from asthma, probably does not have a need for oxygen treatment. Such a casualty should not have oxygen administered to him by those who find themselves in possession of the requisite apparatus, especially if the administration of oxygen is carried out in place of proper and correct first-aid procedures.

GIVING OXYGEN IN FIRST-AID

> In giving oxygen, care must be taken to see that
> —the airway remains clear, and
> —the mask fits.

Oxygen must be given by way of a well-fitting mask, so that the casualty inhales a high concentration of oxygen through the nose and/or mouth. The mask must therefore cover the nose and the mouth. A good fit is very difficult to obtain with people who have no teeth.

A plastic oxygen therapy mask is probably best in first-aid. Anaesthetic-type face masks must be skilfully used in order to produce an airtight seal round the nose and mouth of the casualty by downward pressure, while at the same time keeping the neck extended and the jaw forward to prevent obstructed breathing. We would not recommend the use of anaesthetic-type masks in first-aid unless special training has been given to those who may use the masks. The same would apply to any apparatus which contains an anaesthetic-type mask as a part, such as certain mechanical respirators.

The flow rate to the mask should be 4 litres of oxygen per minute (*Figure 1.7*).

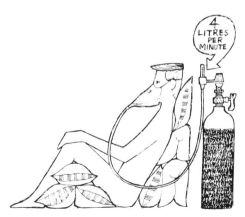

Figure 1.7.—Giving oxygen. Note the position of the casualty which helps difficult breathing

When oxygen is given for blueness, the casualty's colour should usually begin to improve fairly quickly if oxygen is going to help. Oxygen should continue to be given to keep the casualty pink. At intervals, try cutting down the amount of oxygen. If the casualty stays pink, however, oxygen can be stopped and supplies conserved. If, however, the blueness begins to return, continue to give oxygen. If, after giving oxygen for about 2 minutes (30–40 breaths), the casualty's colour does not improve, the use of oxygen is ineffective and should therefore be stopped.

There are some remarks on the use of automatic breathing machines in first-aid on page 246 which are related to the use of oxygen in first-aid.

BEWARE

Giving oxygen is only a partial remedy for inadequate ventilation (breathing). *Airway clearance* is vital and always comes *first* in attempting to deal with breathing difficulties. Correct posture to aid breathing is also very important—for example, the half sitting position, leaning forwards or leaning backwards, as shown on page 104; and the correct use of the unconscious position *lying on the injured side,* in the case of chest injuries.

So, in addition to giving oxygen, other forms of assistance in terms of airway clearance and correct posture to aid breathing will always be required.

a warning about oxygen and the fire hazard

Oxygen presents a serious fire hazard.

Combustion in the presence of high concentrations of oxygen is much more vigorous than in the presence of air which contains about 20 per cent of oxygen. In high-oxygen atmospheres, glowing or smouldering objects such as a cigarette will burst into flame, and anything which is burning will burn much more rapidly and fiercely.

Before turning on an oxygen supply to give oxygen to a casualty, make sure that the safety rules are being followed.

—No sources of ignition such as open fires or naked flames should be present near the casualty or near the oxygen supply.

—No smoking is allowed in the area.

Last, a word of warning about oxygen cylinders— no grease or oil should ever be used on or near the valve, the outlet, or other working part of the cylinder or oxygen apparatus. Nor should these be handled with greasy or oily hands in case the grease or oil is deposited onto the cylinder or valve. Grease or oil may ignite spontaneously in the presence of oxygen with disastrous consequences to all concerned. Stiff valves on oxygen cylinders should NEVER be lubricated; such cylinders should be screwed tightly *shut* and should be returned to the supplier with a label attached saying 'stiff valve'.

CHAPTER 2

BLEEDING AND BLOOD LOSS

All injuries cause some bleeding and serious, especially multiple, injuries cause serious bleeding.

P. S. LONDON, FRCS

MEDICAL INFORMATION

INTRODUCTION

In order to understand the mechanisms of bleeding and of blood loss, it is useful to begin by considering the general effects of injury. These general effects, sometimes called 'shock', can best be described and reviewed in first-aid by considering injuries in which no vital structures or important organs are damaged. We are here distinguishing between the *local* tissue damage which occurs at the site of an injury and the *general effects* of that injury on the injured person.

The general effects of injury

In limb injuries in man, that is, in injuries in which no special vital organ is damaged, the general effects of injury have been shown to be brought about by various combinations of

—blood loss

—tissue damage

—nervous disturbance such as pain and fright.

In the early stages of limb injury, that is, at the stage at which the first-aider will normally see the casualty, *the only major factor producing general effects is blood loss*. Good first-aid can stop external bleeding quickly, can recognize internal bleeding, and can set priorities with regard to the need for blood replacement.

In the case of tissue damage, good first-aid can make sure that the damage does not become worse, by careful handling of the injury and of the casualty. In the third category, nervous disturbance, the casualty can be comforted and reassured by sympathy tempered by tact.

But by far the most important cause of general effects of injury where no vital organ or structure is damaged is *bleeding*.

Kinds of bleeding

Bleeding may arise from arteries, from veins or from the very small blood vessels, the capillaries, which carry blood through nearly all the tissues.

Blood coming from an *artery* may come out in regular spurts in rhythm with the heart beats, or in a gush if the artery is large. If the torn artery is at the bottom of a deep wound, however, the blood will not spurt out but will flow out of the filled cavity of the wound. As the blood in arteries is flowing with a higher pressure than elsewhere, more blood is lost more quickly by arterial bleeding than by venous or capillary bleeding.

Blood in *veins* is at a much lower pressure and will flow or trickle out. The amount of flow will depend on the size of the vein, the extent of the damage to the vein and whether the blood flow is aided by downhill flow (down from the heart) or prevented by uphill flow (for example, by lifting up a leg in a person who is lying down and thus getting the bleeding part higher than the heart). Varicose veins are often large and bleed easily and freely.

Bleeding from *very small blood vessels* ('capillary bleeding') will depend on the size of the wound.

It is not generally of importance in first-aid to distinguish between these various forms of bleeding. Bleeding should be stopped by pressing where the blood comes from, by limb elevation and by rest. Blood loss should be replaced in hospital—SOON.

NORMAL BLOOD VOLUME

Table 2.1 gives the approximate normal blood volumes.

In children blood volumes are closely related to weight—about 70 ml per kg (1 pint per stone) of body-weight is a rule of thumb approximation. In adults, height gives a better rough guide, tall people having more blood.

TABLE 2.1

Age *(years)*	*Blood volume*	
	(millilitres)	*(pints, approximately)*
At birth	300	Just *over* $\frac{1}{2}$
$\frac{1}{2}$	500	Just *under* 1
1	700	Under $1\frac{1}{2}$
3–5	1,250	Just *over* 2
10	2,800	Just *under* 5
20	4,370	About $7\frac{3}{4}$
Average adult female	4,370	About $7\frac{3}{4}$
Average adult male	5,500	About $9\frac{3}{4}$

BLOOD LOSS FROM THE CIRCULATION

Blood, to be of use to the body, must remain in circulation. Blood loss is the amount of blood which *is lost to the circulation*, regardless of whether the blood is lost to the *outside* of the body through wounds—by external bleeding—or whether the blood is lost *inside* the body, for example, around a broken thigh or within a body cavity such as the chest or abdomen—by internal bleeding.

Pooling of blood is, in addition to bleeding, a means by which blood can be lost to the circulation. The muscular walls of small blood vessels can become lax and as a result the vessels fill with blood. If this happens on a large scale, as it may do, then a large amount of blood is pooled in these dilated blood vessels and does not circulate. It could be said that it is even possible to 'lose' half of the circulating volume in this way, under certain conditions.

In discussing blood loss, we should be concerned with two important facts.

(*i*) The *actual amount* of blood which represents the normal blood volume for that individual.

(*ii*) The *proportion* or fraction of that normal volume *which is not circulating*.

The actual amount of blood which represents the normal blood volume for an individual is the standard against which any loss must be measured. For example, a loss of 250 ml of blood in a fit adult will not be a significant loss, but in a child aged 6 months this represents half of the total blood volume and would thus be very serious indeed. In discussing proportions or fractions of blood lost, related to normal blood volumes, we shall always speak in *twelfths*. It is possible to relate the severity or nature of certain injuries to the anticipated blood loss arising from the injury, and to express this in twelfths of the total blood volume. It is also possible to relate known spills to fractions of the estimated blood volume and thus to assess the severity of the blood loss. The details of this are given on pages 42–46.

Adults can lose from the circulation up to about 2/12 of their total blood volume without any very serious effect on their general condition. A loss of 3/12 of the circulating volume will give rise to moderate general effects. Any loss of over half, that is, 6/12, of the circulating volume is likely to be fatal unless blood replacement is swiftly carried out. Children and old people tolerate blood loss less well than adults.

critical reserves

There is a certain amount of any tissue or organ—including blood—which can be lost without affecting the

33

capacity of the body as a whole to survive the loss. But there is also a *critical reserve*, that is,

> the minimal amount of any tissue or organ which is compatible with survival.

Blood, which consists of a fluid—plasma—in which the red and white blood cells are carried, can be thought of in three ways for the purpose of discussing critical reserves.

	Critical reserve
Whole blood	8/12
Red cells	4/12
Plasma	8/12

In the case of *whole blood* a sustained loss of more than 4/12 of the initial volume is critical. Initially, this effect is due simply to *fluid depletion*. A sustained loss of 4/12 or more of whole blood can lead to death because there is then no fluid reserve to draw on. Fluid replacement is therefore *a matter of urgency* (*see* intravenous infusions, page 58).

Intravenous replacement by blood is, of course, the treatment of choice in whole blood loss. However, if this cannot be done, intravenous plasma, plasma expanders, or intravenous saline solution or glucose–saline solution can be used to replace the fluid loss until whole blood is available.

In the case of *red cells*, the critical reserve is 4/12 of the initial volume. Whole blood loss will therefore present problems of fluid loss before giving rise to problems of oxygen transport due to lack of red cells.

If *plasma loss* is the problem—resulting from burns, for example—intravenous replacement by plasma is the treatment of choice. However, if whole blood, plasma or plasma expanders are not available, intravenous fluid replacement by saline solution or glucose–saline solution can be used until blood or plasma become available.

Fluids by mouth may be useful as a first-aid measure, particularly in the case of burns. If drinks are taken too quickly, vomiting may ensue, thus increasing fluid loss. Fluids should therefore be given slowly and frequently, *in sips,* not gulps. The quantities given should not exceed half a cup every 10 minutes or so in an adult, timed by a clock—write it down. Personal estimation is notoriously unreliable. Children will require less in proportion to size. Remember, NO fluid should be given to unconscious persons.

THE GENERAL RESPONSE OF THE BODY TO BLOOD LOSS

The response of the body to blood loss will depend on three things
—the rate of bleeding, that is, whether the blood loss is fast or slow; fast blood loss requires fast replacement;
—the volume (amount) of blood which is lost from the circulation;
—whether blood loss is, or is not, associated with other serious conditions.

We all know that in most cases a healthy adult can give one bottle of blood slowly without any ill effect. Occasionally, there may be a slight tendency to feel faint, dizzy or light-headed for a few minutes only. The amount of blood lost in such circumstances is usually not more than about 1/12 of the total blood volume.

When blood is lost from the circulation, the body attempts to make the best use of existing blood by
shutting down the blood supply to non-essential areas, and increasing the rate of circulation.
—shutting down the blood supply to non-essential areas;
—increasing the rate of circulation;
—mobilizing blood and fluid from within the body.

Shutting down the blood supply to non-essential areas, such as the skin, takes place in order to maintain circulation to essential areas such as the brain, heart and lungs. It is this shutting down of circulation to the skin which gives rise to the characteristic appearance and findings in a casualty who has bled. He is pale, with the pallor affecting the skin and the

35

lips. The palm of the hand is often a good guide to colour. The skin is cold and clammy to touch and the casualty feels that it is cold. The shutting down procedure also helps to maintain blood pressure.

Increasing the rate of circulation usually occurs when bleeding in excess of about 3/12 of normal volume takes place.

General changes with bleeding

These changes are summarized in Table 2.2.

TABLE 2.2

	Blood loss		
	Slight (about 2/12 of normal blood volume)	Moderate (3/12 to 4/12 of normal blood volume)	Severe (over 4/12 of normal blood volume)
General condition	Not much affected	Affected Anxious	Very poor Anxious and restless
Colour	Pink or slightly pale	Pale	Very pale or bluish
Temperature of hands and feet	Warm	Sometimes warm, sometimes cold	More often cold
Pulse rate	Normal, low or slightly raised	Normal or raised	Raised
Pulse volume	Normal or high	Normal	Low

The general condition is a good guide to moderate bleeding.—The general condition of any casualty who bleeds will tend to get worse with increasing blood loss until he becomes limp, pale, perhaps unconscious, and eventually pulseless and lifeless from extreme blood loss. There is often a stage where the casualty appears to be holding up generally in a very encouraging way in spite of known severe blood loss (say, 4/12–5/12). At this stage, the casualty can only be hanging on to the brink of a precipice by tremendous effort—all his emergency mechanisms are mobilized and working to full capacity. Any further strain, however slight, sets the stage for total collapse.

In severe bleeding collapse may occur.—The casualty becomes pale, cold and limp, the pulse is rapid and feeble, breathing is sighing in character and consciousness may be clouded or unconsciousness may supervene.

Giddiness, faintness, ringing in the ears, a feeling of incipient black-out and finally loss of consciousness may show that the brain is not getting enough oxygen from the blood (cerebral anoxia).

We should, therefore, in first-aid, remember that the treatment for blood loss is blood replacement—SOON—and try to recognize that any casualty who has lost over 3/12, that is, one-quarter, of his blood volume is heading for the precipice of collapse, and that any casualty who has lost over 4/12, that is, one-third, of his blood volume is hanging on the edge. Only swift arrest of bleeding and rapid blood replacement by transfusion will take such a casualty away from the brink of collapse and death.

Therefore, if you know that a casualty has lost a dangerous amount of blood, even if he appears well, do not be misled into thinking that there is no urgency in the situation. He may collapse at any time. Your job is to do what is necessary to maintain life and prevent deterioration, leaving undone anything else, and get him to hospital quickly for blood replacement.

Pallor increases with blood loss.—Slight blueness may also be present and is best seen in the edges of the ear, in the lips, at the tip of the nose and in the nail-beds. If you have any doubt about colour—either pallor or blueness—compare the colour of your own skin and nail-beds with that of the casualty, or look at the colour of any bystanders. Sometimes, under poor lighting, it is very difficult to recognize colour changes—

so remember to carry a good torch in your first-aid kit or car to enable you to compare the casualty's colour with another normal person's if you can, or with your own.

The hands and feet grow cold and surface veins are empty.—As more blood is diverted from the skin and from the limbs to keep essential body organs, including the heart, lungs and brain, supplied with blood, the extremities—the hands and feet—grow cold and clammy due to absence of blood supply. This condition does not usually appear until bleeding has been more than moderate (3/12) in amount. The surface veins on the back of the hands may be seen to be collapsed and empty of blood under these conditions.

Pulse changes with bleeding

As severe bleeding goes on, the heart will tend to beat faster. This is because, as blood cells are lost, the oxygen-carrying capacity of the blood will diminish, unless the rate of circulation of cells is speeded up. By speeding up the rate of circulation, one cell can be made to do more oxygen-carrying than previously.

An analogy might be to think of lorries delivering units of oxygen. To deliver 10 units of oxygen every hour, 4 lorries going at an average speed of 20 mph are normally required. But the same delivery rate of 10 units per hour may be achieved by 3 lorries travelling at 27 mph or 2 lorries at 40 mph. The speed of the circulation will tend to rise with the blood loss because the need to deliver oxygen around the body will remain about the same.

Therefore, the rate of the heart beat, taken by counting the pulse beats per minute, will be fastest with greatest blood loss and less fast with a smaller blood loss. Another way of saying the same thing is that *the rise in pulse rate will tend to be proportional to the amount of blood loss* until collapse sets in due to excessive blood loss.

As the pulse rate rises, the change in the rate can be measured against time. The faster the pulse rate rises, the

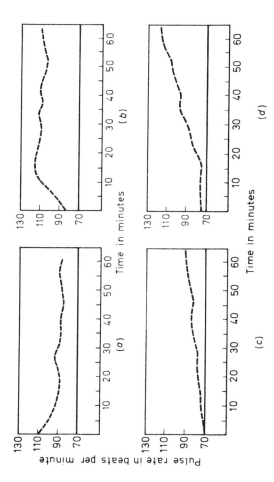

Figure 2.1.—(a) An excited casualty who had some slight blood loss but is not bleeding now. (b) Fairly rapid blood loss of at least a moderate amount, followed by no further blood loss. (c) Moderate continuing bleeding; check carefully for external blood loss—if none is found the bleeding must be internal. (b) Bleeding internally and continuously with no sign of stopping. Hospital treatment urgently required.

quicker and more severe is the bleeding. *The speed of rise of the pulse rate when measured against time is a valuable indicator of the amount and speed of blood loss.* This is specially important in internal bleeding. Some examples of pulse charts in bleeding are given in *Figure 2.1.*

The pulse volume, which is the amount of blood moved by each heart beat, *will fall as bleeding proceeds*, and the pulse will change from a normal full pulse to a feeble, thin and thready one.

HOW TO RECOGNIZE AND ASSESS THE AMOUNT OF BLOOD LOSS FROM THE CIRCULATION

Be aware that bleeding may take place and look for bleeding

It may seem to some readers a rather strange fact that people have bled to death without this being recognized until they are dead. This state of affairs is bad enough in internal bleeding where the blood cannot be seen, though of course the condition can be recognized. However, if the bleeding is external, one would expect that the bleeding would be recognized and treated. It is because external bleeding is *not always recognized* and treated that it is necessary to begin this section by saying that unless the casualty is examined initially for possible bleeding by looking at the back as well as at the front, and is subsequently watched for recurrence of bleeding or for fresh bleeding, lives will continue to be lost. For example, an obvious wound on the head of an unconscious casualty may be treated, while he bleeds away his last remaining blood from a serious wound behind the knee which has cut through the artery.

Bleeding must be carefully looked for, *especially underneath the casualty*, or it may not be found.

A check on the general condition of the casualty, plus a pulse record *written down* at 5-minute intervals should allow any bleeding to be recognized. It may be appropriate to quote here the old adage that 'more things are missed by not looking than by not knowing'.

Spilling

An attempt should always be made to assess the volume (amount) of blood which can be seen. A little practice with any sticky fluid on the floor will soon lead to well-informed guesses about the amount lost. For example, a spill on a flat surface of 0·6 × 0·3 metre (2 × 1 feet) would amount to about 300 ml (about half a pint). This amount would soak about half of a skirt.

Soaking

Blood will be soaked into clothing and dressings. Again, the amount of staining and *dampness* will give a clue to the volume of blood lost. Always feel underneath a casualty for dampness. *Any dampness felt must be assumed to be due to bleeding until proved otherwise* by close inspection. Such inspection may necessitate removal or cutting of clothing.

General condition

As bleeding proceeds, the general condition gets worse *and the casualty looks ill.* Beginning with slight pallor and dizziness or a feeling of weakness, the condition proceeds by stages of coldness, further weakness, anxiety, faintness and marked pallor, to collapse with urgent long-drawn sighing breathing, slight blueness and terminal unconsciousness, and then to death. Careful observation of the casualty at any stage will disclose the general condition.

How to look for and recognize severe bleeding

Note skin colour carefully, and look at the tips of the ears and the nail-beds for any sign of blueness. Feel the skin—is it hot or cold, dry, slightly clammy or distinctly moist? Does the casualty appear pale, tired and weak, with a feeling of dizziness and coldness; is he unconscious, or is the general condition that of a normal alert responsive person? Restlessness and nausea may occur. Extreme bleeding can cause unconsciousness. Any casualty who has lost 3/12 or more of his total blood volume will always look ill, so

41

examine casualties carefully and check their general appearance as well as the detail of their injuries.

Restlessness may be an important indication of bleeding.

In the absence of severe pain, restlessness usually means marked and progressive bleeding.

This fact is well worth remembering when faced with a restless casualty who is not in pain; internal bleeding may be occurring. Even with pain present, restlessness should always lead the first-aider to think about bleeding.

Disproportion between *apparent injuries* (slight) and the *general condition* of the casualty (poor) may often be an indicator of internal bleeding. For example, a casualty was seen suffering from a closed fracture of one wrist and recovering from slight concussion, but he looked ill. The general condition was worse than would be suggested by these injuries. More detailed questioning about how the injury happened revealed that the casualty had suffered a heavy blow with some crushing on the right lower chest and upper abdomen. Further examination of the casualty showed that there was tenderness over this area. Internal bleeding from a ruptured liver could therefore be suspected as the cause of the casualty's poor general condition, and other signs of internal bleeding such as a rising pulse rate could be sought on the way to hospital.

Estimate the volume of blood loss by the injuries sustained

It is possible to predict the probable amount of blood loss which will result from any particular injury. Soft tissue injuries, the size of the casualty's hand spread out, may lose 1/12 of normal blood volume. Deep soft tissue injuries should be compared with the casualty's fist—one fist-sized wound may lose 1/12 of normal blood volume. *Figure 2.2* gives details. By adding together the numbers appropriate to each injury, the amount of blood loss in twelfths of normal total blood volume can be estimated. In this way the severity

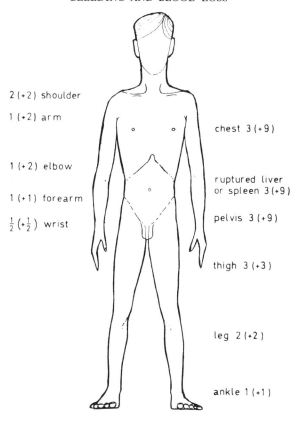

2 (+2) shoulder

1 (+2) arm

chest 3 (+9)

1 (+2) elbow

ruptured liver
or spleen 3 (+9)

1 (+1) forearm

pelvis 3 (+9)

$\frac{1}{2}$ $\left(+\frac{1}{2}\right)$ wrist

thigh 3 (+3)

leg 2 (+2)

ankle 1 (+1)

Figure 2.2.—A guide to blood loss from fractures, wounds or injuries of various regions. The first figure is the amount which is usually lost; the figure in parentheses is the amount of additional blood which may be lost. All figures are in twelfths of normal blood volume. In the case of open fractures, add 1 or 2. Add spillage or soaking. One hand-sized surface wound counts as 1; one fist-sized deep wound counts as 1; any count over 4 means that more than 4/12 of the casualty's blood volume has been lost to the circulation and there is need for blood replacement soon.

of blood loss can be estimated and the need for blood replacement gauged. It is also useful in assessing the general condition of the casualty against the known injuries. These should be comparable; if not, why?

For example, a casualty may have a fracture of the leg (2), fracture of the forearm (1) and a fist-sized deep wound in the thigh (1). He will thus have a predicted blood loss of 4/12 of his normal blood volume, which means that there is need for blood replacement soon.

Any casualty who has lost

slight amounts	up to 2/12 of blood volume	*may* need blood transfusion
moderate amounts	3/12 to 4/12 of blood volume	*will* need blood transfusion soon
severe amounts	over 4/12 of blood volume	*must* have blood transfusion urgently

The blood volumes, as on page 32 are repeated in Table 2.3, together with the amounts which represent slight, moderate and severe blood loss.

It should also be remembered when assessing the severity of blood loss that children and old people are less able to withstand blood loss than fit young adults. Therefore, smaller amounts of blood loss will cause more severe general effects and will be more threatening to life in children and old people. The loss of 650 ml of blood, as can be seen from Table 2.3 is a slight loss in an adult, a moderate loss in a child aged 10 years or over, and a severe loss in a child aged 5 years.

Pulse changes

We would emphasize the need to

FEEL
MEASURE and
WRITE DOWN
at frequent
intervals
⎱ the *pulse rate* and the *actual time*, in all cases of bleeding or suspected bleeding.

44

TABLE 2.3

Age (years)	Blood volume		Blood loss (millilitres)		
	(milli-litres)	(pints, approxi-mately)	Slight (about 2/12 of normal blood volume)	Moderate (3/12 to 4/12 of normal blood volume)	Severe (over 4/12 of normal blood volume)
At birth	300	Over $\frac{1}{2}$	50	75–100	100+
$\frac{1}{2}$	500	Under 1	85	125–165	165+
1	700	$1\frac{1}{3}$	115	175–235	235+
3–5	1,250	Over 2	210	310–415	415+
10	2,800	Under 5	415	625–835	835+
20	4,370	$7\frac{3}{4}$	730	1,090–1,455	1,455+
			May need blood transfusion	Will need blood transfusion soon	Must have blood transfusion urgently
Average adult female	4,370	$7\frac{3}{4}$	730	1,000–1,500	1,500+
Average adult male	5,500	$9\frac{3}{4}$	915	1,400–1,800	1,800+

A note should also be made of whether the pulse was weak or strong. If internal bleeding is suspected or is present, the pulse rate, recorded every 5 minutes, will be of enormous help to the doctors in hospital in determining what to do for the casualty. Therefore:

> any casualty who is thought to be bleeding, who is in danger of bleeding or who is known to be bleeding, should have the pulse rate written down at 5-minute intervals until he reaches hospital. It may also be of help to the doctor in hospital to note whether the pulse rhythm was regular or irregular.

Swelling

The initial swelling of a bruise, of a sprain, or around a broken bone is usually due to bleeding, that is, to blood loss from the circulation. All these swellings are due to internal bleeding. The amount of the swelling is, in the early stages, nearly always directly proportional to the blood loss. The more blood lost to the circulation, the greater will be the swelling.

Always compare one side of the body with the other when possible, and compare the injured side with the normal side. People vary in shape and size, and it is often possible to assess the exact amount of swelling by comparing an injured side or part of the body with the uninjured one.

THE APPEARANCE OF BLOOD FROM DIFFERENT PARTS OF THE BODY

Blood from wounds

Everyone is familiar with the bright red blood which is seen from small wounds. In large wounds, lumps of liver-coloured material, which is clotted blood, may also be seen. These clots should not, of course, be scooped out or removed, as this may increase or restart bleeding. Dressings should go on top of the clot.

Blood from the mouth

Blood from the mouth may be mixed with saliva (spit). When the amount of bleeding is small, the usual appearance is streaks of blood in the saliva. In large amounts, the saliva is stained bright red.

The above refers to bleeding which *arises* in the mouth. Blood which *appears* in the mouth may come from:
—the mouth,
—the nose, draining into the mouth,
—the throat,
—the stomach (by vomiting) or
—the back of the throat or lungs (by coughing).
Remember that a fracture of the base of the skull can cause

bleeding at the back of the throat, and this blood may be seen in the mouth.

Vomited blood

Bleeding which causes vomiting of blood may arise from

—*the mouth*. Blood is swallowed and later vomited.

—*the back of the nose, throat or gullet* (oesophagus). Blood is swallowed and later vomited. Occasionally such blood may come from a fracture of the base of the skull.

—*the stomach or duodenum*. The casualty often suffers from known ulcers or indigestion. Abdominal injury may also be a cause.

Fresh blood

When bleeding is fast and vomiting occurs soon, the blood will appear as fresh blood—bright red, and often with liver-like clots.

Digested blood

Digested blood does not look like blood at all, but looks like coffee grounds—small black or dark brown specks in a light brown liquid. Regurgitated digested blood is often referred to as a 'coffee-ground vomit'. When blood stays in the stomach, digestion of the blood begins, and produces this coffee-ground appearance. Only a little of the blood from the stomach may appear in the mouth; most of the blood may go into the intestine, where it is digested and passes out in the motion to give it a black tarry appearance.

Coughed-up blood (from the lungs)

Coughed-up blood appears as bright red *frothy* blood, being mixed with frothy mucus from the lungs. The blood and mucus become frothy because of the air movement through them, thus causing bubbles to form.

If there is any doubt about the origin of blood which appears in the mouth, look in the mouth and throat for any source of bleeding, and ask the casualty whether the blood was coughed up, or was vomited. This information, plus the appearance of the blood and other information, perhaps of a chest injury or a history of indigestion, should explain the source of blood.

Always keep any specimens of blood and vomit to send to hospital with the casualty.

Blood in the stool

Two kinds of bleeding have to be distinguished.

(a) *Fresh blood*

Fresh blood in the stool will appear as bright red blood and will be due to some condition in the lower part of the large bowel, in the rectum or at the anus. The blood will appear as a streaking of bright red on the outside of the motion and on the toilet tissue. Very occasionally, with a large amount of bleeding which has collected in the rectum, clots may be seen.

(b) *Digested blood*

Digested blood makes the stool very dark or tarry black in colour. Bleeding in this case has taken place higher up the gut, for example, in the stomach or duodenum, and the blood has passed through the intestine, being digested as it goes. The motion may thus be normal in one part and black in another—the black segment showing the bleeding which has taken place. Black stools are not usually passed until about 6–8 hours after bleeding from the stomach or duodenum, and may take considerably longer. Such bleeding can of course be recognized when it occurs by faintness, dizziness and pallor, and a rising or raised pulse rate—the signs of concealed internal bleeding—associated perhaps with a history of indigestion.

Blood in urine

Blood in urine in small amounts turns the urine cloudy or smoky in appearance instead of clear. With slightly larger amounts an orange colour may be seen in the cloudy urine. With still larger amounts, the appearance will be bright red and suggests blood. Small clots may also be found.

Any casualty who has had an injury to the kidney region, the loin, the back, the lower abdomen, or the pelvic region, should always have the next specimen of urine kept for examination by a doctor.

Vaginal bleeding

Three kinds of vaginal bleeding can be described.

(*a*) Menstrual bleeding.

(*b*) Bleeding which is not menstrual in a non-pregnant woman.

(*c*) Bleeding in a pregnant woman,
in early pregnancy (up to $3\frac{1}{2}$ months)
in late pregnancy (7–9 months).

These various kinds of bleeding sometimes can be distinguished by taking a careful history of how and when the bleeding came on in relation to normal menstruation and the possibility of pregnancy.

The AIMS of FIRST-AID for BLEEDING

(1) Stop bleeding quickly.

(2) Send the casualty to hospital without delay in case blood replacement is required.

How to stop external bleeding is one of the commonest problems of first-aid, and is usually dealt with by pressure, preferably using a wound dressing over the bleeding area, by limb elevation and by rest. Then send the casualty to hospital.

Bleeding ceases naturally because blood stops flowing and forms a clot. Thus, any measure which encourages blood to stop flowing and to form a clot will stop bleeding, and conversely, anything which encourages flow or breaks up or damages a clot will encourage or allow bleeding to continue.

The first-aid for a casualty with internal bleeding is to put him at rest by making him lie down, and then send him swiftly to hospital. Raise the legs and apply a head-down tip unless the casualty's general condition is very good, or other injuries do not allow this to be done.

Always remember that *blood loss requires blood replacement—soon.*

THE HEAD-DOWN POSITION WITH RAISED LEGS

Any casualty who is thought to be bleeding internally, who has lost more than very slight amounts of blood, and whose injuries permit, should be placed with a head-down tip to keep available blood circulating to the brain, heart and lungs. Similarly, the legs should be raised to mobilize all unused reserves of blood so that this spare blood can be used to best advantage. *These simple measures can be of great value to the casualty, particularly if bleeding has been severe. They are not, in general, used sufficiently often. These measures can be life-saving after severe bleeding.*

PACKING LARGE WOUNDS

Sufficient pressure cannot be applied to stop bleeding from raw surfaces in some large wounds unless the wound is *packed*, that is, the dead space in the wound is filled up with dressing material which is pressed into the space and then built up above the surrounding skin level. Before the encircling bandage is applied—and a *crêpe* bandage is best— the packing material in the wound should extend *well above* the surrounding skin level *(Figure 2.3)*. If the pack material is not protruding above the surrounding skin level, the encircling bandage cannot press the pack downwards into the dead space of the wound to exert pressure on the damaged blood vessels, and thus stop the bleeding.

FIXING THE LIMBS IN MAJOR SOFT-TISSUE WOUNDS

Resting the injured part is an important measure. It encourages the formation of blood clot as a part of stopping bleeding, and prevents breaking up of existing clot.

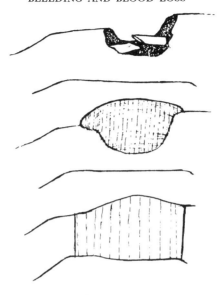

Figure 2.3.—Packing a wound

In order to encourage rest, and to prevent movement which may break up a clot, it is wise to treat any serious or moderate wound in the same way as if there were a fracture of that region. For example, slings can be used in the upper limbs, and the legs may be tied together.

THE FIRST-AID TREATMENT OF VAGINAL BLEEDING
Bleeding which is not menstrual in a non-pregnant woman

Any slight bleeding which occurs in a non-pregnant woman should be treated at home by bed rest and calling the doctor. If the casualty is not at home, or if bleeding is other than slight, the casualty should be treated as a case of visible internal bleeding—keep a pulse chart, and send to hospital. No attempt should be made to plug the vagina. An external pad should be used to absorb the blood.

Bleeding in a pregnant woman

A pregnant woman can be defined for first-aid purposes as any woman of childbearing age who has missed a menstrual period or whose period is overdue.

Two sorts of bleeding may occur.

—Bleeding during early pregnancy (up to $3\frac{1}{2}$ months).

—Bleeding during late pregnancy (7–9 months).

Bleeding during early pregnancy (up to $3\frac{1}{2}$ months).—This sort of bleeding is usually due to an incipient or actual miscarriage (abortion), and occurs most commonly at about the third month of pregnancy.

Strict bed rest and calling the doctor is the appropriate first-aid for cases which occur at home, and who have very slight blood loss. Until the doctor arrives a pulse chart should be kept, and the first-aider should remain with the casualty. Undue excitement in such cases can be helped by a calm manner in dealing with the problem.

If blood loss following a sudden miscarriage is other than very slight in amount, the casualty should be sent swiftly to hospital, following the usual treatment for visible internal bleeding. A pulse chart should be kept during the journey to hospital. No attempt should be made to plug the vagina. An external pad should be used to absorb the blood.

Bleeding during late pregnancy (7–9 months).—This kind of bleeding is usually preceded by occasional very small leaks of blood which give rise to 'spotting' of underwear by blood, and may progress to obvious bleeding. The home first-aid treatment of such vaginal bleeding, if very slight in amount, is to put the casualty to bed and to call the doctor. If bleeding occurs away from home or if it is other than very slight, send the casualty to hospital, treating her in the usual way for visible internal bleeding and making a pulse chart *en route*. No attempt should be made to plug the vagina. An external pad should be used to absorb blood.

Tubal pregnancy (ectopic pregnancy)

While on the subject of bleeding and pregnancy, we should like to digress slightly and to mention here the internal bleeding which can occur from a tubal pregnancy. In some cases, the fertilized egg (ovum) starts to grow, not in the uterus (womb), but in one of the tubes which connect the ovary to the uterus. The tube is not designed to accommodate a growing fetus, and at about the third month the tube may tear due to the enlarging fetus. This tear can give rise to massive and severe internal bleeding. Any woman, who may be about 2–3 months pregnant and who had abdominal pain followed by collapse, should be suspected of having internal bleeding. Start a pulse chart (page 38) at once. Ectopic pregnancy causing bleeding is a potentially life-threatening condition. The treatment is to send the casualty swiftly to hospital so that she can be given blood replacement, soon, and can have an operation to stop the bleeding.

BLEEDING, HEAD INJURIES AND THE PULSE RATE

Particular care should be taken in any casualty who is unconscious following a head injury to look for bleeding, because if bleeding is unrecognized it will not be treated and the casualty may die. Never assume that unconsciousness is due to a head injury, or is the result of excessive bleeding, until you have made a quick general examination of the casualty, a special examination of the head, and have measured the pulse rate. These three, together with a history of what happened—if this is available—will help to make a reasoned diagnosis.

One very special problem may arise.

Severe bleeding makes the pulse rate rise and the pulse volume fall.

Brain compression makes the pulse rate fall and the pulse volume rise.

53

Therefore, a casualty who has a head injury with brain compression and who is also bleeding—say, internally—may have a pulse rate and volume which may tend to mislead the first-aider. For example, if the rise in pulse rate due to internal bleeding is matched by an equal fall in the rate due to brain compression, the pulse rate remains the same although the general condition of the casualty is getting very much worse.

It is only by knowing that this paradoxical effect can arise, and by looking at the general condition of the casualty and recognizing deepening of unconsciousness, increased pallor and worsening of the general condition that the contradictory effects of these two conditions on the pulse rate can be recognized. Therefore:

(i) always check all unconscious casualties very carefully for bleeding.

(ii) always check any casualty, whom you think may be unconscious due to blood loss, for signs of head injury (unequal pupils; wounds or bumps on the head; blood or straw coloured fluid (cerebrospinal fluid, page 70) from the ears, nose, mouth or throat).

(iii) remember that the pulse rate should be recorded at 5 minute intervals. If brain compression and bleeding are both present the pulse rate may be an unreliable guide.

(iv) if both brain compression and blood loss are suspected, or have taken place, the casualty must reach hospital in as short a time as is possible, consistent with carrying out essential first-aid and not injuring the casualty further by an unnecessarily rough journey.

See again page 75 for a discussion of the effects of brain compression on the pulse rate, and page 38 for the effect of bleeding on the pulse rate.

WHY TOURNIQUETS AND RUBBER BANDAGES ARE TO BE AVOIDED IN FIRST-AID

Tourniquets and rubber bandages as a means of stopping bleeding are more often misused than properly used. In addition, they carry dangers of cutting off blood supplies to areas which need blood. Lastly, and this may seem strange, both tourniquets and rubber bandages can cause increased bleeding. A personal experience may make this clear.

A man was found at the edge of a road having suffered an amputation of his leg midway between the knee and the ankle. A rubber bandage had been applied round the remains of the calf. There was a noticeable flow of blood from the severed end. Release of the rubber bandage immediately lessened the flow of blood and light pressure over the stump stopped the bleeding completely. Elevation was not necessary.

Why did release of the constriction lessen blood flow and why did this simple pressure on the stump stop the bleeding completely when a constricting bandage did not?

To answer these questions, it is necessary to understand that blood flowing down the leg in arteries is at a pressure of, for example, about 100 mmHg, or above. Return blood flow in veins is at a much lower pressure of about 5 mmHg or less (Hg = mercury).

If an encircling rubber bandage is applied at a pressure of more than 100 mmHg, that is, at a pressure higher than the arterial pressure, blood flow in the arteries down the leg will cease. Blood flow in the veins will also stop completely, below the encircling bandage *(Figure 2.4)*.

However, if the bandage is applied at a pressure of *less* than 100 mmHg, blood flow down the leg *will not* be stopped, but blood flow back up the leg from all points beyond the constriction *will* be stopped *(Figure 2.5)*. The effect of such 'treatment' is to increase blood loss, because any blood which flows down the leg past the constriction cannot get back. Pressure in the blood vessels beyond the constriction

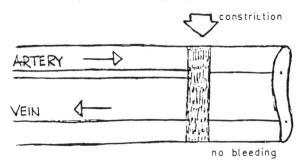

Figure 2.4.—Constriction at a pressure greater than the pressure of the blood in the artery and in the vein: blocks *blood flow* downwards in artery; blocks *blood flow* upwards in vein—*resulting in NO BLEEDING but may endanger tissue which is below the constriction because the* blood supply is cut off

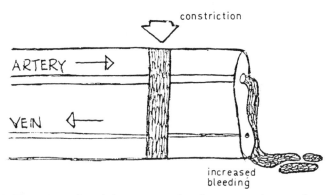

Figure 2.5.—Constriction at pressure less than artery and greater than vein: permits *blood flow* downwards in artery; blocks *blood flow* upwards in vein—*resulting in INCREASED BLEEDING and all the risks of blood loss, and DANGER to all tissue below the constriction because blood may not circulate*

will rise due to inability of the blood to flow back past the constriction. The only pressure relief in such a system is by blood draining outwards from damaged blood vessels, thus becoming lost to the body. This was the situation in the casualty quoted above.

Figure 2.6 shows why the methods of stopping external bleeding by pressing where the blood comes from and by elevation are best.

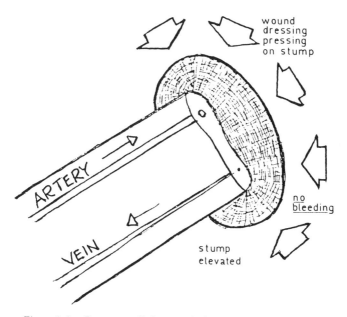

wound
dressing
pressing
on stump

ARTERY

VEIN

no
bleeding

stump
elevated

Figure 2.6.—Pressure applied over end of stump; stump elevated. No constriction of artery or vein: permits *blood flow through the* artery; permits *blood flow through the* vein—*resulting in NO BLEEDING and NO DANGER TO TISSUES*

INTRAVENOUS INFUSIONS ('DRIPS')

There are three main forms of intravenous infusions which may be of use in first-aid.

  (i) Saline solution or glucose–saline solution.

 (ii) Plasma or plasma-expanders.

(iii) Whole blood.

These intravenous infusions should only be given under the direction of a doctor. It is not, therefore, our intention to discuss the techniques of intravenous infusions, but to give some idea of the possible uses of each, by way of background interest for the first-aider.

Saline solution or glucose–saline solution

Saline solution or glucose–saline solution will be given to replace fluid loss quickly, especially where fluids by mouth may be difficult or dangerous. Possible examples where they would be used in the treatment of hyperpyrexia *(salt/fluid depletion)*, and following prolonged vomiting associated with seasickness or with a diarrhoea–vomiting type of illness. It may also be useful in the early stages of burns of moderate severity or worse if plasma is not available, and following bleeding of 4/12 or more of normal blood volume, to replace fluid if whole blood is not immediately available.

Plasma or plasma-expanders

The principal use of plasma—or plasma-expanders if blood plasma is not available—will be following burns of moderate severity or worse. In general, adults with burns of 18 per cent or over of body surface should be considered as possibly requiring a plasma infusion, and over 25 per cent should certainly have plasma infusion started as soon as is practicable after injury (page 158). Children and old people will require plasma with lesser areas of burning. Young children with 10 per cent burns will probably require plasma. The general condition of the casualty should also be taken into consideration in assessing the need for plasma. Plasma or plasma-expanders may also be used to replace the fluid loss following severe bleeding until whole blood becomes available.

Blood

Any casualty who has bled more than 2/12 of his blood volume *may* require a transfusion. Losses of 3/12 and over *will* require to be replaced, and losses of over 4/12 *must* be replaced soon or urgently. Whole blood is the transfusion of choice following blood loss.

CHAPTER 3

INJURIES

PREVENTION

Careful investigations which have been made into the causes of injuries occurring at home, at work or on the roads, show that *most injuries can very easily be prevented*. It is the exceptional case in which preventive action—usually simple—could not have been applied.

The treatment of injuries, whether by first-aid, home treatment or in hospital, is always a poor second to prevention.

THE CAUSES OF INCIDENTS

In order to prevent injuries, it is necessary to have some idea about the many causes which led to each injury. For example, a heavy weight may fall unexpectedly. This could lead to injuries *(Figure 3.1)*, or it could lead to damage

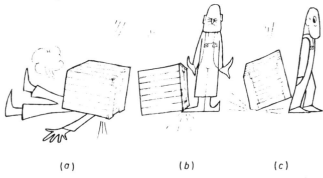

(a)   (b)   (c)

Figure 3.1.—Injuries from a falling block. (a) A fatal or serious injury;
(b) a minor injury; (c) no injury

(Figure 3.2). Various combinations of injury and damage could also occur. The *critical event* in each case is the same—a heavy weight falls unexpectedly—but once the weight starts to fall, it is CHANCE which determines the consequences.

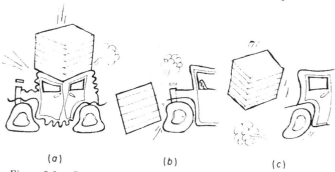

(a) (b) (c)

Figure 3.2.—*Damage from a falling block. (a) Catastrophic or serious damage; (b) minor damage; (c) no damage*

Therefore, preventive effort, to be effective, must be applied BEFORE the critical event, in this case before the weight falls.

The events outlined above could be summarized as in *Figure 3.3.*

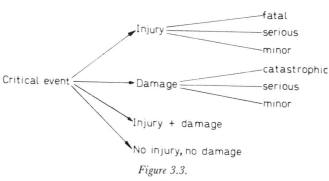

Figure 3.3.

Similarly, if a car went suddenly out of control, the result could be

—nothing; the driver regains control and goes on.

—no injury but serious damage; the driver escapes injury, but the car is badly damaged.

—serious injury and slight damage; the driver falls out of the vehicle as it rolls over and is badly hurt, but there is only slight damage to the vehicle.

—fatal injury and serious damage; the driver is killed and the vehicle is badly damaged.

The critical event

In each example, the critical event was constant, but was followed by different consequences. CHANCE determined the consequences. So, if we are to prevent injuries we must look before the critical event—the weight falling or the car going out of control. It is only when we understand WHY the critical event took place that we can apply successful preventive action.

We should *not* assume that all is well because the critical event in any particular instance results in neither injury nor damage. Indeed, this result is a friendly but urgent warning; the consequences *by chance* have been nothing, but could easily *by chance* have been fatal injury or serious damage. An opportunity for preventive action has been highlighted. Whether it is taken or ignored will depend on how aware we are of the true significance of the incident.

People and things

If we continue to use the two examples above, and ask why the critical event took place, in the case of the weight falling, there may, for example, have been failure of the suspending wire, or mechanical failure of a crane (environmental causes: unsafe conditions); or there may have been inattention or improper operating procedures on the part of the crane operator (personal causes: unsafe acts); or there may have been a combination of these conditions, for example, improper operating procedure, inattention leading to mechanical failure of the crane and severance of the suspending wire.

In the case of the car going out of control, a front tyre may have punctured suddenly, again why—was it a good tyre, did the driver knowingly use a bad tyre, and so on; or there may have been a patch of oil on the road; or the driver, having had a lot to drink, was driving too fast on a wet road in a car with defective brakes.

In general terms, part of causation can be described as having to do with *people* and part to do with *things*. The results of investigations into a large number of incidents in which *all* causes were investigated and assessed have shown that

> *the important causes of injury and damage are to do with PEOPLE in three-quarters of the incidents and to do with things in a quarter of cases.*

Put another way, this says that *human behaviour is the most important cause in the majority of human injuries*. If we are to influence the pattern of injuries by prevention, then in most cases we have to influence people and their behaviour, and in a smaller number of cases we have to look to the environment.

This lesson is hardly appreciated by many people. It is always much easier to blame things than to face the unpleasant reality that *people*—oneself or one's friends and acquaintances—have behaved unsafely. It is all too easy to shrug off dangerous acts which result in no serious consequence, but the fact remains that we have to influence people and their behaviour in the majority of incidents if preventive action is to become effective.

All this should not minimize the need to look also at *things,* or the need to attend to the safety of our environment— attention here is vital. However, many people already know and accept this part of the picture but are not so aware or appreciative of the important part which human behaviour plays in the causation of *most* of the incidents which result in injury or damage.

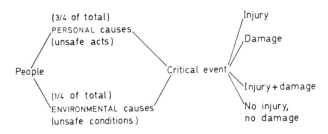

Figure 3.4.

The complete sequence of causal events, whether at home, on the roads, or at work, could be shown as in *Figure 3.4*. It should be noted that the word 'people' appears at the front of the chart. Unsafe acts are carried out by people, and unsafe conditions are created by people. In a similar way, *safe* conditions could be created by people.

Conclusion

The application of prevention should follow logically from an understanding of causation, and must be applied *before* the critical event takes place in order to be effective.

Our preventive efforts tend to be directed more to things than to people. Without minimizing our present efforts, we must increasingly study and apply the methods by which human behaviour can be influenced—by education, leadership, training, discipline, propaganda, example, exhortation and so on, and weigh up the effectiveness of each method in any situation in order to prevent injuries and damage. In this way, we shall be more successful.

HEAD INJURIES

Head injuries will be discussed in two main groups.
   —head injuries in which there is brain damage.
   —head injuries without brain damage.

HEAD INJURIES WITH BRAIN DAMAGE

Some common ways of sustaining brain damage are
—to hit the road with the head due to a fall from a motor
   cycle.
—to be flung out of a car in a car crash.
—to hit the head on the roof of a car after an impact.
—to fall from a height on to the head.
—to have an object strike the head.
—to become unconscious for some reason and then to fall,
   striking the head.

THE PREVENTION OF INJURIES WHICH CAUSE BRAIN
   DAMAGE

   Most injuries, including head injuries, are of a preventable kind. Hard hats could be worn more generally, for
example in many sports such as horse riding, when their
use would undoubtedly prevent some serious injuries.

   In industry, hard hats though increasingly worn are still
not to be seen in many situations where they would undoubtedly be useful, or are worn by only a proportion of
the work force.

   Many people who could be saved from serious injury die
every day in car crashes because they are flung out of the
car or because they strike their head or chest against parts
of the car. A seat belt, if fitted and *worn*, could save many of
these lives. It would also prevent crippling long-term
injuries which result in permanent disability. The evidence
in favour of seat belts being fitted and worn is now beyond
any *reasonable* doubt.

Knowledge, to be useful, must be applied. Example is a powerful stimulus to others. Here is where a knowledge of the consequences of head injuries can be used to try to increase the preventive action which can be taken, so as to avert the many needless head injuries which occur every day.

MEDICAL INFORMATION

NORMAL BRAIN FUNCTION AND BRAIN DAMAGE

In first-aid, it is often necessary to decide whether a head injury has been accompanied by brain damage. The indications that the brain has sustained damage may be any or all of the following.

—Any change whatever from normal full alertness.

—Loss of memory for recent events.

—Loss of sensation (numbness) of any part of the body.

—Loss of movement (paralysis) of any part of the body.

—A head wound with a depressed fracture.

—Any wound which opens the skull.

—Bleeding from the ear, nose or back of the throat and mouth.

—Bruising behind the ear.

—Cerebrospinal fluid (a clear, watery liquid) leaking from the ear, nose or back of the throat and mouth.

—Unequal pupils or pupils which do not react to light.

—A black eye.

—Epileptic attacks or uncontrolled movements of arms and/or legs.

—Odd or curious behaviour of any kind.

—Anyone who cannot reply to questions *in sentences.*

Any change from normal full alertness.—This is *by far* the most important indication of brain damage. The possible changes in the level of consciousness may be thought of as every shade of grey from white (full normal alertness, fully

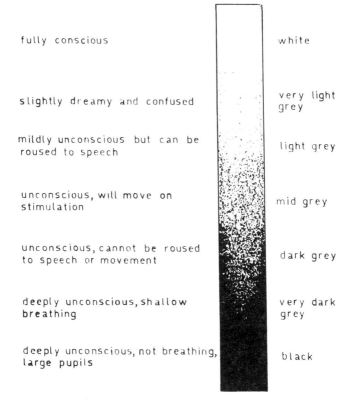

fully conscious — white

slightly dreamy and confused — very light grey

mildly unconscious but can be roused to speech — light grey

unconscious, will move on stimulation — mid grey

unconscious, cannot be roused to speech or movement — dark grey

deeply unconscious, shallow breathing — very dark grey

deeply unconscious, not breathing, large pupils — black

Figure 3.5.

conscious) to black (unconscious, unrousable and not breathing). The range of possibilities is therefore considerable and is through a continuous scale. This is illustrated in *Figure 3.5.*

It is thus possible to pick out and to name various points— but the scale is really a continuous one. When reviewing

67

any case of loss of consciousness, whether due to head injury or to another cause, the first-aider will want to know whether the loss of consciousness came on suddenly or slowly, whether the casualty is becoming more or less conscious—going up or down the scale, or remaining the same—and the rate of any change. Another way of putting this is to say that the first-aider will want to know:

(1) *the level of consciousness,* and
(2) *any change in the level of consciousness measured against time,* and whether the change is fast or slow, upwards or downwards.

A small series of diagrams *(Figure 3.6)* will help to illustrate these points.

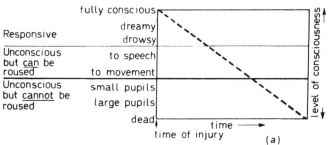

Figure 3.6. (a) *Progressive loss of consciousness worsening all the time.*

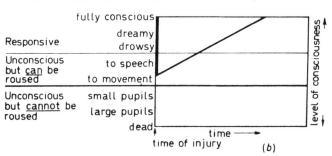

Figure 3.6. (b) *Sudden loss of consciousness and then improvement to normal.*

68

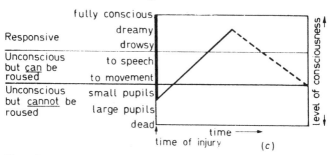

Figure 3.6. (c) Sudden loss of consciousness followed by improvement at first and later by worsening.

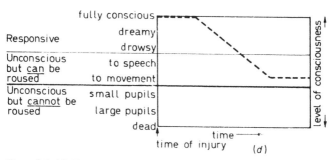

Figure 3.6. (d) Normal full consciousness and then progressive loss of consciousness with levelling off.

Loss of memory for recent events.—Casualties who have suffered a head injury often show a loss of memory for events which immediately preceded the injury. For example, a man may be found having fallen from his bicycle. He appears to be fully conscious and co-operative and has a small bump on the head. He does not remember any loss of

69

consciousness and nobody saw him immediately after his fall. Did he in fact have any brain damage? Close enquiry may reveal that he remembered leaving home, but that he cannot remember cycling the last quarter of a mile, although everything was clearly remembered until then. He cannot give any account of why he fell off his bike, and therefore shows loss of memory. This sort of evidence should always be sought. It is often much more gross than this example and may involve not knowing the day of the week and not remembering getting up, dressing, having breakfast or leaving home and cycling. As time passes, however, events begin to be recalled, starting in the past and finishing just short of the events which led up to the injury.

Loss of sensation (numbness) or loss of movement (paralysis) of any part of the body.—These will indicate damage to the brain, spinal cord or to the nerves which go out to the affected part. Tingling of 'pins and needles' may herald loss of sensation in a part of the body.

A head wound with a depressed fracture.—A depressed fracture may press on underlying brain. Bleeding as a result of the injury may also damage the brain. This bleeding can arise

(a) from damage to the arteries which run along the inside of the skull,

(b) from damage to blood vessels in the brain covering, or

(c) from damage to blood vessels within the brain itself.

In every case, the result of the bleeding will be to press on brain substance, thus injuring the brain (*see Figure 3.9*).

Any wound which opens the skull.—Such wounds may damage the brain and may also cause bleeding within the skull.

Bleeding or leaking of cerebrospinal fluid from the ear, nose or back of the throat and mouth.—These are signs that the skull, and therefore the brain, may be severely damaged. If there is no obvious local cause for bleeding, then the blood must be coming from inside. Cerebrospinal fluid (C.S.F.), which is a clear, watery and sometimes straw-coloured fluid, can come only from inside. Any violence which can cause leaking of blood or C.S.F. from inside is enough to damage the brain. Blood and C.S.F. may be mixed, resulting in a watery looking type of bleeding. Always look for C.S.F. alone, or mixed with blood, from the nose, ears and throat in casualties who have head injuries or who are unconscious. A C.S.F. leak means also that bacteria could gain access to the areas where the fluid comes from, thus giving rise to meningitis or other serious infection.

Unequal pupils or pupils which do not react to light.—Three things should be noted about the pupils in all cases of known or suspected head injuries.

(*a*) The actual size of the pupils.

(*b*) Whether the pupils are of the same or different sizes, that is, whether they are *equal* or *unequal* in size.

   The best way to record the size of the pupils is to draw on a piece of paper a circle which corresponds to the size of the pupil. Always remember to indicate the right eye, left eye and the time.

O   O

Left eye   right eye 1730 hours

   Such notes should be repeated at intervals so that change or absence of change in pupil size can be noted, with times.

(*c*) Whether or not the pupils *react to light*.

   In order to find out whether the pupils react to light, the eyes should first be shaded and the lids closed. After about 5 to 10 seconds the eyelid(s) should be opened or raised, and a bright torch or light should be shone into the eye. A normal eye reacts immediately,

71

and the pupil gets smaller. A sluggish reaction indicates some damage, and no reaction indicates worse damage. Each eye should be tested separately, and the observation should be made twice on each eye if the reaction is not normal.

In general, as a casualty becomes increasingly unconscious, the eye signs will be as in Table 3.1.

TABLE 3.1

Degree of unconsciousness	Eye signs
Drowsy	The lids tend to close The lids close
Unconscious but rousable (sleep)	The eyeballs move from side to side, the so-called 'roving eye'
Unconscious, cannot be roused	The eyeballs stop moving. They then remain looking straight ahead. At this point the pupils are small in size
Very deeply unconscious	The pupils grow larger
Nearly dead	The pupils become fully enlarged

In cases of head injury, if the pupils are unequal, the injured side will *usually* have the larger pupil, and the larger pupil will be the one which does not react to light.

In looking for eye signs, beware of the casualty with the glass eye. Even doctors have made mistakes here!

A black eye.—All black eyes should be seen by a doctor because they may be due to a fracture of the skull or they may result in serious damage to the eye (page 116). In the context of head injuries, a black eye should always be associated with the possibility of a fracture of the skull—and this with bleeding within the skull causing brain damage.

Epileptic attacks or uncontrolled movements of arms and/or legs.—An epileptic attack or fit can be described simply as an alteration of consciousness, which may be anything from slight drowsiness to unconsciousness, accompanied by un-controlled or twitching movements of the arms and/or legs. The face and body may also be involved in these uncontrolled movements. (*See* page 187 for further information about epilepsy.)

Odd or curious behaviour of any kind.—Any curious or bizarre behaviour which follows a head injury must be presumed, in first-aid, to be due to brain damage.

After a head injury, some casualties may appear truculent and may refuse to go to hospital. It is important to make allowances for the behaviour being due to injury, and to treat the casualty as someone who is not himself, who *will* require hospital treatment. Persistance and firmness may be required on the part of the first-aider in order to get the casualty safely delivered to hospital!

THE CLASSIFICATION OF BRAIN DAMAGE

Brain damage following injury can be classified thus.
(1) Concussion.
(2) Compression, from bleeding inside the skull.
(3) Localized brain damage from wounding.

Concussion

Concussion *(Figure 3.7)* is the name given to a particular type of brain injury which is characterized by:
(*i*) immediate onset.
(*ii*) steady recovery from the time of onset of recovery.
(*iii*) being produced by rapid acceleration or deceleration of the head. The injury producing force tends to be a blunt force which causes sudden movement or sudden arrest of movement of the head, or both.
(*iv*) damage throughout the substance of the brain. The damage is not localized to the point of impact.

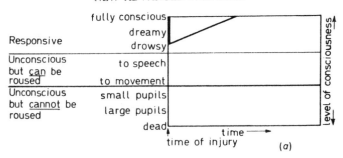

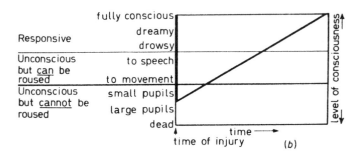

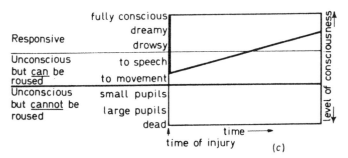

Figure 3.7.—Three examples of concussion. (a) Mild concussion with rapid recovery; (b) severe concussion with slower recovery; (c) moderate concussion with slow recovery

Compression (bleeding inside the skull)

Compression *(Figure 3.8)* of the brain by bleeding inside the skull is a life-threatening emergency, the treatment for which is to open the skull, relieve the pressure on the brain and stop the bleeding. In normal circumstances this is only done in hospital.

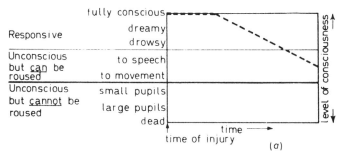

Figures 3.8. Examples of compression. (a) Slow bleeding; compression effects do not show for some time after the injury; steady deterioration of the level of consciousness.

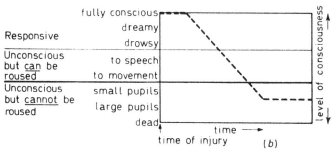

Figure 3.8. Examples of compression. (b) More rapid bleeding; fast deterioration of the level of consciousness; bleeding stops and level of consciousness steadies out.

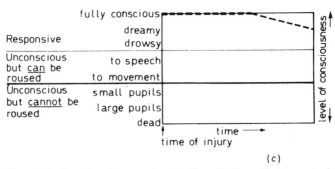

Figure 3.8. Examples of compression. (c) Slow bleeding with late onset of change in level of consciousness; very easily missed unless casualties with head injuries are observed regularly for some time after the injury.

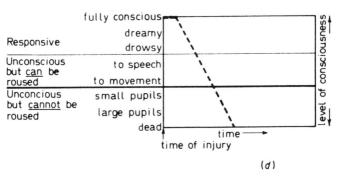

Figure 3.8. Examples of compression. (d) Rapid bleeding with swift deterioration of level of consciousness; operation must be swift in order to save life; speed in getting the casualty to hospital makes the difference between life and death.

How to recognize that bleeding is occurring inside the skull.—
(*i*) By the kind of injury.
(*ii*) By a downward trend in the level of consciousness.
(*iii*) By a *slowing* of the pulse rate.

76

by the kind of injury.—In *any* head injury, including mild ones, the possibility of bleeding inside the skull should always be borne in mind. Any head injury which gives rise to loss of consciousness or to a fractured skull, especially to a depressed fracture, or to severe headache, should always be sent swiftly and comfortably to hospital in case bleeding takes place inside the skull. Remember that if there is any possibility of brain damage, the casualty should always be sent to hospital. Skull radiographs may be required.

by a downward trend in the level of consciousness (see Figure 3.9)

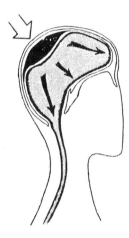

Figure 3.9.—*Blood may compress the brain*

by a slowing of the pulse rate.—This sign will only be found if it is looked for. The pulse rate should be *written down* at 5-minute intervals, together with the actual time of the observation. As compression of the brain due to bleeding proceeds, the base of the brain is wedged into the hole at the base of the skull through which the spinal cord passes

(Figure 3.9). When the base of the brain stem is compressed, the heart rate slows. The pulse therefore feels of good volume —not feeble—and becomes *slower* as the compression proceeds.

The combination of a pulse which is slowing with a continuing downward trend in the level of consciousness means bleeding inside the skull which is causing compression of the brain. This condition must be recognized at the earliest possible moment so that the casualty can be sent swiftly but gently and without delay to hospital.

It should be noted that the volume of blood which is required to produce a pressure rise inside the skull is *small* in amount. Therefore, the casualty will *not* show signs of blood loss from the circulation as in other forms of internal bleeding. There will not be a rising, feeble pulse.

Brain compression leads to a slowing of the pulse rate and the blood loss to a quickening of the pulse rate. Thus, difficulty may arise in interpreting the pulse chart in casualties with brain compression who are bleeding elsewhere. The resolution of this paradox is fully discussed on pages 54 and 55 in the chapter on bleeding.

Concussion and compression may occur together or one after the other in the order concussion, then compression, but never the other way round. This is a common sequence of events following motor cycle crashes, where the pillion rider is flung off and his head hits the road. There is a sudden deceleration when his head strikes the road which results in concussion. Later, bleeding inside the skull leads to brain compression. Depending on the time relationship between recovery from concussion and the downward effects on level of consciousness from compression, there may be no recovery from unconsciousness (*Figure 3.10(a)*—severe concussion, slow recovery, swift bleeding leading to compression), or there may be apparent complete recovery from

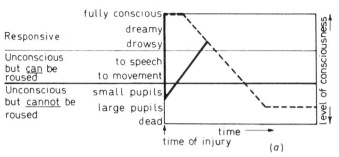

Figure 3.10. (a) *Fairly severe* concussion. *Onset of compression masked by depth of unconsciousness due to concussion; change in direction from recovery to deepening unconsciousness due to* compression; *bleeding stops and level of consciousness steadies out.*

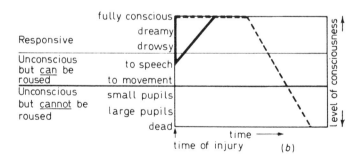

Figure 3.10. (b) *Moderate* concussion. *Apparent complete recovery; slow* bleeding, *leading eventually to* compression; *fatal outcome.*

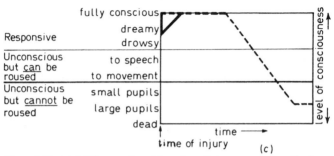

Figure 3.10. (c) Mild concussion. Apparent complete recovery; slow bleeding, leading to compression: bleeding stops and level of consciousness steadies out.

concussion *(Figure 3.10(b))* followed by increasing drowsiness and unconsciousness, and even by death if the downward trend in level of consciousness is not recognized and immediate action taken.

> A downward trend in the level of consciousness which follows a previous upward trend is a sign of bleeding inside the skull giving rise to brain compression. If this compression is not swiftly relieved, the casualty may die.

The events which are shown in *Figure 3.10(c)* happened to a cyclist. He was riding home late at night on a bumpy road, hit a stone and came off. He was sitting by the side of the road, shaking his head and feeling a bit dizzy, when a neighbour pulled up in his car and asked if he could give him a lift. The cyclist declined the offer with thanks, saying that he felt all right and, having only a short distance to go, could easily ride home on his bike. The neighbour, to be on the safe side, drove slowly behind him and saw him enter his house. Soon after his arrival, the cyclist complained of a headache, took two aspirins and went straight to bed. The next morning, some 7 hours later, he did not respond to a call. He was found to be deeply unconscious. The moral of this is that anyone who has had, or is suspected of having had, a head injury should be observed for 4–6 hours after the injury to detect any change in the level of consciousness in a downward direction after apparent recovery. If such casualties are not spoken to hourly, any deterioration in their condition may not be discovered until much later than it could have been. In any case of doubt about a head injury or suspected head injury, the best course of action is to take the casualty to hospital.

Localized brain damage from wounding

Localized brain damage from wounding is the least common cause of brain injury. We are here disregarding any general effects of such injuries and considering only the localized damage to the brain which occurs, for example, along the track of a penetrating injury or at the site of a skull fracture. The effects of local brain injury will depend on which part of the brain is injured.

The AIMS of FIRST-AID for HEAD INJURIES

(1) Treat for unconsciousness, if present.
(2) Prevent infection.
(3) Record (that is, write down) the level of unconsciousness or consciousness and the pulse rate at 5-minute intervals until the casualty reaches hospital.
(4) Send the casualty to hospital, watching and recording *en route*.

TREAT FOR UNCONSCIOUSNESS

The main points are: remove dentures, debris and loose or broken natural teeth; remove any blood or vomit from the back of the throat by mopping with a handkerchief or paper tissue, or, if possible, by the use of a sucker; turn the casualty into the unconscious position with a slight head-down tip. If there is blood coming from one ear, this side should be downwards. Check breathing carefully and stay with the casualty—unconscious casualties must never be left alone.

PREVENT INFECTION

The types of head injury which tend to have problems due to infection are head wounds with a depressed fracture, and casualties in which there has been bleeding or leaking of blood or C.S.F. from the ear, nose, mouth or from the back of the throat and mouth (see page 47).

Cover any head wounds.—Use a sterile dressing if possible, or the cleanest dressing available, but remember, do not press on any head wound in case there is a fracture of the skull and bone is thus pressed on to the brain. Handle all head wounds very gently, and handle the whole head carefully in the presence of brain or head injury. Use pads or above-ear encircling bands to stop bleeding.

Instruct the casualty **not** *to blow his nose.*—Blowing the nose in the presence of skull fractures or facial injuries may, by back pressure, carry infection into remote spaces or force air through cracks into the inside of the skull or elsewhere where the presence of air can be dangerous.

Any nasal discharge should be carefully examined for the presence of blood and/or cerebrospinal fluid, and should be wiped away, not blown out.

MAKE RECORDS

The importance of a clear account of what happened at the scene of injury, of what the condition of the casualty was when first seen, and of the subsequent course of the casualty's condition is most useful to enable correct treatment to be carried out when the casualty reaches hospital.

Records should include times of observation of all facts and should be *written down*. People cannot remember things clearly. Changes in the level of consciousness or pulse rate cannot be clearly assessed without a written record of the level of consciousness and the pulse rate *and* of the actual time.

It is for reasons such as these that a sharpened pencil or a ball-point pen and supply of writing paper in pad form should be a part of every first-aid kit!

SEND THE CASUALTY TO HOSPITAL

Any casualty who has suffered a head injury with loss of consciousness should be sent to hospital. He should be observed carefully during the journey for any deterioration in the level of consciousness.

—Fully conscious head injury casualties should travel in the position which they find most comfortable to them.

—Semi-conscious head injury casualties should be placed in the unconscious position without a pillow, and should have dentures removed in case they become unconscious.

—Unconscious head injury casualties should be placed in the unconscious position with a slight head-down tip, following the rules for the treatment of unconsciousness.

Any head injury casualty who is thought to be bleeding inside the skull, and is showing signs of compression such as a fall in the level of consciousness and a slowing pulse, should be taken to hospital as quickly and gently as possible so that the brain compression can be relieved.

A message should also be sent by radio—most ambulances are fitted with radio—or by telephone to the hospital to tell them that, for example, a casualty will be arriving suffering from suspected bleeding inside the skull causing brain compression. In this way, everything will be ready to deal with this emergency on arrival in hospital.

A careful watch should be kept on the casualty at all times. All observations should be written down. Watch especially for obstructed breathing.

Head injuries plus serious injuries elsewhere

The association of head injuries with serious injuries elsewhere must always be remembered. Many head injury casualties are unconscious and therefore cannot complain of pain at the site of other injuries. Broken arms or legs, dislocated shoulders, elbows or hips, chest injuries, fractures of the pelvis, abdominal injuries and spinal injuries must all be looked for and treated appropriately.

Priorities in the management of multiple injuries will be to
  (*i*) deal at once with obstructed or difficult breathing, and with severe bleeding.
 (*ii*) recognize quickly any rapid fall in the level of consciousness and to send the casualty swiftly to hospital.
(*iii*) deal with fractures, dislocations and minor wounds if required or if appropriate.

We have mentioned individual priorities again at this point because proper assessment of injuries is the key to individual priorities. Always examine unconscious casualties for other injuries.

When priorities are established serious injuries which *must* be treated in order to save life can be differentiated from other injuries which are not life-threatening. The less serious injuries must therefore be left untreated in order to get a seriously injured casualty to hospital for treatment of the serious and life-threatening injuries. Skilled neglect of unimportant injuries and correct priorities in treatment will save lives.

Unconsciousness in the presence of a head injury is not always due to the head injury

A casualty who has an obvious head injury and is unconscious is not of necessity unconscious *due to* brain damage from the head injury. The casualty may, for example, have had a stroke or a heart attack, or may be suffering from airway obstruction, insulin overdosage, poisoning or internal bleeding. All of these may cause unconsciousness; the head injury may be a secondary feature.

A word of warning

>   *Morphine or pethidine should NOT be given to casualties who have a head injury or suspected injury.*

Notes on the use of morphine and pethidine in injured casualties are given on pages 138–142. Attention is again drawn to the need to withhold morphine and pethidine from casualties who have head injuries with brain damage or from casualties who are suspected of having brain damage.

Self-help in head injuries

Stopping bleeding and summoning help are probably the first priorities in self-help. These will follow the usual procedures. If dizziness and faintness occur, or you think that you may lose consciousness, lie down in the unconscious position, loosen tight clothing at the neck and remove any dentures.

A 'knock-out'

A 'knock-out' is an example of brain injury produced by rapid acceleration or deceleration of the head—in other words, the casualty suffers from *concussion*.

THE WHYS OF THE TREATMENT OF UNCONSCIOUSNESS

We have said a great deal both here and elsewhere about how to treat unconsciousness without giving the whys, except in an indirect way *(Figure 3.11(a))*. What follows is an explanation of the reasons for treating unconsciousness in the way we do.

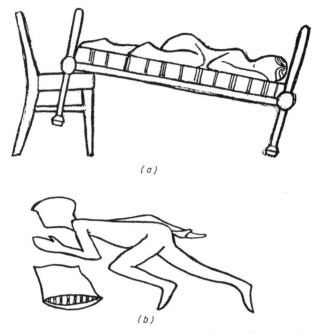

(a)

(b)

*Figure 3.11.—(a) Lift the bottom of the bed. (b) The unconscious
position—do not use a pillow*

We have already written about the need for a clear airway
in unconscious casualties and have drawn attention to the
20 per cent or more of people who die from inability to
breathe because of airway obstruction. This alone is justifi-
cation enough for the treatment which is outlined. At a
later stage in time, however, the commonest cause of death
in head injury cases with unconsciousness, who survive the
immediate brain damage, is pneumonia. The pneumonia is
caused by inhalation of secretions or vomit while the
casualty is unconscious. This pneumonia which frequently
leads to the death of the casualty is, in the majority of cases,

preventable by properly applied first-aid. But, when pneumonia has occurred, it is difficult to treat in spite of antibiotics and other modern treatment.

Here again is a situation in which any first-aider can prevent the onset of a potentially fatal condition by applying the simple treatment for unconsciousness.

The reasons for the use of the unconscious position with a head-down tip *(Figure 3.11(b))* are therefore

(1) to prevent airway obstruction or partial obstruction, and

(2) to prevent inhalation or syphonage of secretion and vomit. Any secretion, blood or vomit will flow *out* of any casualty who is in the unconscious position *with a head-down tip*.

Saliva, vomit or blood in the mouth, nose or throat of any unconscious casualty lying on his back will drain into his lungs and will tend to obstruct his air passages. Similarly, fluid which is pooled in the pharynx may be sucked or syphoned into the air passages and lungs. The only safe course of action is to place all semi-conscious and un-conscious casualties in the unconscious position with a head-down tip and full neck extension to keep the airway clear *(Figure 3.12)*. *Never* wait for gurgling noises indicative of, and resulting from, obstruction and possible inhalation of secretions before doing so. Similarly, in the case of vomiting,

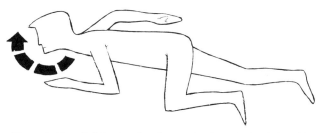

Figure 3.12.—Full head and neck extension in teeth-clenched position to keep airways clear

it is too late to act effectively if the casualty has vomited while lying on his back. The only really safe thing to do is always to turn the casualty into the unconscious position with a head-down tip *before* he can vomit.

A SYNOPSIS OF IMPORTANT POINTS ABOUT HEAD INJURIES WITH BRAIN DAMAGE

—The amount of recovery which is possible from any particular head injury is often determined largely by the quality of the early treatment. First-aid is a very important part of early treatment.

—Always treat unconsciousness correctly and swiftly and make sure that obstructed breathing cannot occur. If obstructed breathing does occur, recognize and treat it at once. Watch unconscious casualties carefully for any sign of obstructed breathing and NEVER leave them alone.

—In any major head injury, however urgent, always record
  (*i*) the level of consciousness,
  (*ii*) the size of the pupils and
  (*iii*) whether the face, arms and legs can or will move, and any lack of movement (paralysis) found.

—Some do nots:
  (*i*) DO NOT warm or heat any head injury casualty.
  (*ii*) DO NOT give drugs—morphine is particularly dangerous.
  (*iii*) DO NOT give anything by mouth.
  (*iv*) DO NOT leave alone in case obstructed breathing occurs.

—Remember to look for other injuries; unconscious casualties cannot complain of pain and thus guide you to other injuries.

—Do not delay the arrival at hospital of any casualty who has a serious head injury by 'treating' trivialities.

HEAD INJURIES WITHOUT BRAIN DAMAGE

Serious injuries to the face, jaw, nose and mouth can arise from situations in which the face strikes into things or is struck by objects. The most common causes are road traffic injuries, or injury by machinery.

The AIMS of FIRST-AID for INJURIES of the FACE, JAW, NOSE and MOUTH

(*i*) Secure and maintain a clear airway.

(*ii*) Stop any bleeding and cover wounds.

(*iii*) Send the casualty to hospital.

SECURE AND MAINTAIN A CLEAR AIRWAY

In dealing with serious injuries which affect the face, jaw, nose or mouth, the first question must always be 'can the casualty breathe—is the airway clear?'

Pull the jaw and tongue forwards in order to secure a clear airway to the lungs. Conscious casualties will tend to have less difficulty with airway clearance than unconscious casualties. When the jaw has been pulled forward, this will make sure that the tongue will not fall back and block the back of the throat.

An extra careful watch should be kept to make sure that the airway is not obstructed due to movement of the casualty or to further bleeding from injuries.

STOP ANY BLEEDING AND COVER WOUNDS

Injuries to the face and neck region tend to bleed freely. Bleeding can be controlled as usual by pressing where the blood comes from.

Bleeding from the cheek, lip or tongue

The method of applying pressure to the cheek, lip and tongue is to use a gauze swab or other form of dressing and apply pressure to both sides of the area. For example, pressure can be exerted over the lip from *both* inside and outside of the mouth. This method can best be applied by the casualty, after the first-aider has applied the dressing in the correct place. With the aid of a mirror, self-help may be given.

Bleeding inside the mouth

This should be dealt with by pressure in the form of plugs in tooth sockets, or by finger pressure as described above for bleeding from the cheek, lip or tongue. In unconscious casualties make sure that the airway does not become obstructed by blood, and that any small trickle of blood which you cannot staunch escapes outwards from the mouth. Casualties may die from an obstructed airway. They will not die of blood loss from a trickle of blood which escapes from the mouth, provided that they are taken swiftly to hospital.

SEND THE CASUALTY TO HOSPITAL

When you have secured a free airway and have stopped any major bleeding, the casualty should be sent to hospital. During the journey a specially careful watch should be kept to see that the airway remains clear, especially in unconscious casualties.

SOME EXAMPLES OF FIRST-AID

Fractures of the jaw

No bandaging is necessary for fractures of the jaw. If the casualty is conscious he may be allowed to sit up, leaning forwards. The great danger of a fractured jaw, especially in an unconscious casualty, is airway obstruction due either to blood or vomit.

Conscious casualties can help to keep the jaw forward by hooking their index finger over the lower front teeth. Unconscious casualties should be placed in the unconscious position with a head-down tip, and the jaw should be pulled well up and forward to keep the tongue from blocking the airway.

A wound of the tongue

Ask the casualty to put his tongue out as far as it will go. Put a gauze swab over the wound and round the tongue. Tell the casualty to grasp the swab and to pinch the tongue to stop any bleeding. Send to hospital.

A broken nose

There will usually be bleeding from the nose. The casualty should be sent to hospital, holding the nose if necessary. No attempts at all should be made to straighten out a broken nose.

CHEST INJURIES

Chest injuries are serious injuries—and the number of chest injuries which occur is increasing. Some are due to falls from a height, or due to crushing by machinery or earth. Road crashes result in many chest injuries—by crushing or impact, or by being flung out of moving vehicles (*see Figure* 3.12). Quite apart from the need for general preventive measures to reduce road injuries, every driver could help to prevent this injury happening to him by wearing a seat belt. Do you?

Chest injuries seldom occur alone. Of chest injury casualties who were admitted to a hospital in Oxford, 80 per cent had a head injury as well. Limb fractures were found in

NEW ADVANCED FIRST-AID

What happens in a frontal crash

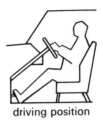

driving position

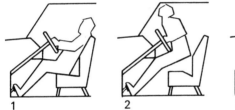

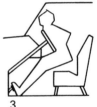

1   2   3

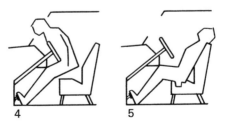

4   5

Note head, chest and knee injuries. Neck and abdominal injuries are also possible.

26 per cent and abdominal injuries in 4 per cent of the chest injury casualties.

Therefore, casualties who have chest injuries are likely also to have head injuries, and vice versa. So, *when either head or chest injuries are found, the other should be looked for especially.*

Chest injuries may be almost impossible to recognize in unconscious, fully-clothed casualties. Even experienced doctors may have difficulty. However, if the story of how the injury happened is sought, if chest injury is suspected, if a careful but swift examination of the chest is made, then chest injuries may be found.

MEDICAL INFORMATION

The chest can be thought of as a bony and muscular cage which encloses the heart and lungs. Serious damage to this cage may result in damage to the heart and lungs.

Damage to the *chest wall* and *lung* may interfere with normal breathing and may make respiration very difficult indeed. In these cases, the experienced and skilled first-aider can accomplish a great deal.

NORMAL BREATHING

In order to understand how chest injuries can affect breathing, it is necessary to know something of how air is normally moved in and out of the lungs.

How air enters the chest and lungs—breathing in

The space inside the chest cavity is made larger by the diaphragm moving downwards and the ribs and chest wall moving outwards and upwards, thus lowering the pressure inside the chest cavity so that air is *sucked in* to fill the space (*Figure 3.13*).

Figure 3.13.—When breathing IN

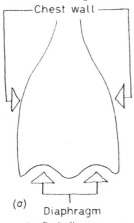

(a)

Diaphragm

(a) *Basic diagram.*

(b) *the diaphragm moves down,*
air enters the chest cavity.

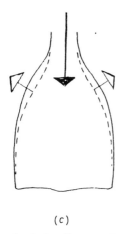

(c)

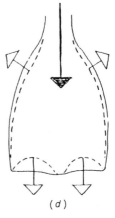

(d)

the chest wall moves outwards,
air enters the chest cavity.

(d) *the diaphragm moves down and the*
chest wall moves out, air enters the chest.

94

How air leaves the chest and lungs—breathing out

The space inside the chest cavity is made smaller, so that air is *pushed out (Figure 3.14)*. We could think of the lungs as

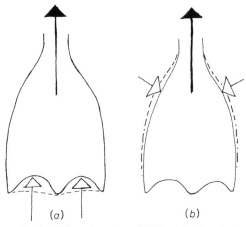

(a)   (b)

Figure 3.14.—When breathing OUT, (a) the diaphragm moves upwards, air leaves the chest; (b) the chest wall moves inwards, air leaves the chest

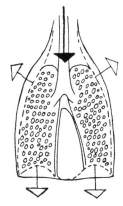

Figure 3.15.—The basic diagram for breathing IN with lungs, trachea and heart added

95

two balloons inside the chest cavity. The lungs are partially separated by the heart *(Figure 3.15)*. The lungs are filled by air as the chest cavity space increases on breathing in. Air leaves the lungs due firstly to contraction of the chest cavity space because the chest walls collapse inwards under their own weight, and secondly to the elasticity of the lungs forcing the air out, like balloons emptying.

It should be noted that in normal breathing
when a person breathes IN the chest and abdomen move OUTWARDS, and
when a person breathes OUT the chest and abdomen move INWARDS.

ABNORMAL BREATHING
Breathing will be impaired if
—there is obstruction to the air passages.
—the respiratory centre in the brain is not working properly.
—there is an open chest wound.
—there is an unstable segment in the chest wall.
—there is bleeding inside the chest cavity.

There is obstruction to the air passages
Obstruction to the air passages is the commonest and most important cause of impaired breathing in first-aid. Obstructed breathing can be due to the jaw sagging and the tongue blocking the airway due to non-use of the unconscious position for an unconscious casualty, or to blood, vomit, dentures, loose natural teeth or debris blocking the airway.

The respiratory centre in the brain is not working properly
The respiratory centre is in the brain stem close to the part of the brain which controls heart beat (page 77). Any-

96

thing which causes damage to this area of the brain will make the control of breathing movements fail—partially or completely. This happens when a casualty is deeply unconscious, for example, as a result of a head injury or following electrocution or poisoning. The part of the brain which should tell the muscles to operate is not working— and so the casualty does not breathe in.

Other examples of conditions which can cause the respiratory centre to fail are serious head injuries which cause brain damage, lack of oxygen reaching the brain, bleeding inside the skull causing brain compression, and bleeding within the brain substance in the area of the respiratory centre.

There is an open wound in the chest

In normal breathing, air is sucked into the lungs, but in the presence of an open chest wound, that is, a wound in

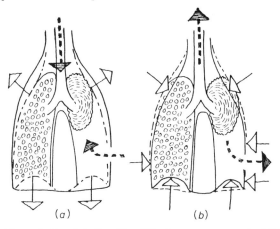

Figure 3.16.—(a) Breathing IN when an open wound of the chest is present. Note collapse of lung and diminished air entry to lung. (b) Breathing OUT when an open wound of the chest is present. Note diminished amount of air leaving the lung

the chest which goes through the wall and into the chest cavity, the air will enter the chest cavity *through the wound* and will occupy the chest space *outside the lung.* The air does not enter through the mouth and nose and will not inflate the lung. Instead, the air will fill the very small space which is normally between the lung and chest wall. The lung on the side of the wound will therefore collapse and will be *deflated* by the air which presses on the outside of it. Therefore the casualty will be unable to breathe normally with this lung because it cannot be fully inflated *(Figure 3.16).*

There is an unstable (flail) segment in the chest wall

An unstable segment can arise when rib damage is extensive. Because it is easier, on attempting to breathe in, to suck an unstable segment inwards than it is to suck air into the lungs, the unstable segment will move in, and the air in the lung will tend to move from one lung to the other rather than in through the mouth and nose. This unstable segment, detached from the normal chest wall and able to move freely and independently from the rest of the chest wall, is often called a 'flail segment' *(Figure 3.17).*

Similarly, it is easier to move the unstable segment outwards than it is to shift air out of the lungs.

Any airway obstruction, by making it more difficult to move air in or out of the chest, will increase movement at the loose and unstable segment and will thus make matters worse. We would therefore emphasize again the importance of keeping the airway clear.

The movement of the unstable segment of chest wall on

breathing *IN* is *INwards,* and on

breathing *OUT* is *OUTwards.*

That is, the movement is contrary to the expected direction of movement of the chest wall when breathing normally (page 99). This phenomenon is known as *paradoxical movement.* Therefore, when paradoxical movement is seen, an unstable segment can be diagnosed. Due to the unstable

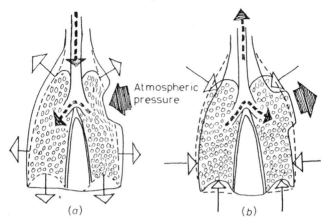

Figure 3.17.—(a) Breathing IN when an unstable segment is present. The unstable segment moves; air entry to the lungs is poor, and air movement takes place between the lungs. (b) Breathing OUT when an unstable segment is present. The unstable segment moves; air exit from the lungs is poor, and air movement takes place between the lungs

segment, air may not pass in and out of the lungs in the required quantity, and the casualty may then show signs of blueness (cyanosis) of the lips and skin, and signs of distressed breathing.

There is bleeding inside the chest cavity

Blood inside the chest cavity will pool and collect at the lowest part of the cavity *(Figure 3.18)*. The lowest part will, of course, depend on the position of the casualty, that is, whether he is sitting or lying. The adjacent lung will be compressed by the blood, and that part of the lung which is compressed will therefore be of no use for breathing. The extent of compression of the lung will depend on

(a) the amount of bleeding into the chest cavity and

(b) the position of the casualty.

99

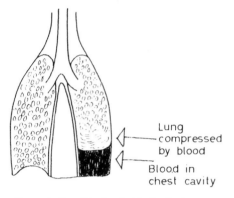

Lung
compressed
by blood

Blood in
chest cavity

Figure 3.18.—Bleeding inside the chest

In chest wall injuries blood which is found in the chest cavity usually comes from bleeding which arises from the inside of the chest wall and not from bleeding which is connected with lung injury.

The AIMS of the FIRST-AID TREATMENT of CHEST INJURIES

(*i*) *Keep the airway clear at all times.*

(*ii*) Convert open chest injuries into closed ones as quickly as possible using an *airtight* seal.

(*iii*) Make sure that the casualty can shift air in and out of the lungs, that is, that he can breathe.

(*iv*) Remove the casualty swiftly to hospital.

KEEP THE AIRWAY CLEAR AT ALL TIMES

A routine check should be made in the mouth for dentures, debris, or loose natural teeth, and for any blood or vomit which may obstruct the back of the mouth and throat. All such obstructing materials should be removed. A handkerchief or cloth may assist in the removal of blood or vomit.

Best of all is a sucker with a soft rubber tube which can be used to suck out any liquid or semi-solid material.

CONVERT OPEN CHEST INJURIES INTO CLOSED ONES

Open chest injuries should be made into closed ones as soon as is possible, *using an airtight seal (Figure 3.19)*. A good airtight seal can be made by using a gauze dressing to cover the wound and then using wide (3 inch) sticking plaster to cover the gauze completely and to seal the edges.

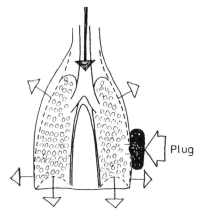

Plug

Figure 3.19.—Breathing IN when the open wound is plugged. Air can enter the lung in normal amounts

An alternative method if no sticking plaster is available is to use a bulky dressing which is damped with water and then tied over the wound with a chest binder. Cling film wrap could also serve in emergency. If nothing else is available, use the casualty's own blood-stained clothing to plug the wound.

The seal should cover an area which is larger than the wound. If you are not sure whether a chest wound is or is not an open wound, always treat the wound as if it is an open wound by applying an airtight seal dressing.

MAKE SURE THAT THE CASUALTY CAN SHIFT AIR IN AND OUT OF THE LUNGS

To make sure that the casualty can shift air in and out of the lungs is neither so easy nor so obvious as it sounds. When there is an unstable segment, air may shift within the chest cavity, that is, from lung to lung, but not necessarily in and out of the lungs.

The pain of fractured ribs and the compression of lung by bleeding within the chest cavity also reduces the ability to shift air in and out of the lungs.

Unstable segments should be recognized by paradoxical movement and by pain. In order to allow the casualty to move air in and out of the chest, it will be necessary to *fix the unstable segment*. Otherwise, the air may move from lung to lung as the unstable segment moves in and out.

Two methods can be used to fix unstable segments.

Self-help or first-help

The casualty can use his own hand to press on the unstable segment and to hold it in at all times *(Figure 3.20)*. When the casualty tries to breathe in, the unstable segment will not be drawn in further because it is already pressed in, and air will therefore be sucked into the lungs. When the casualty tries to breathe out, the unstable segment will not move outwards, and air will be pushed out of the lungs. Less total air will move in and out of the lungs by comparison with normal breathing, but the air will move!

First-help

A pad can be constructed to fit the unstable segment. The pad is then bound to the chest wall to hold the unstable segment in. Use bandages round the chest, or wide sticking plaster 8 cm (3 inch) for this purpose.

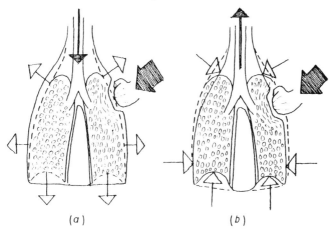

(a)   (b)

Figure 3.20.—Pressure by hand or by pad and binder will stabilize the unstable segment, thus allowing normal air entry and exit to and from the lungs

If, in spite of fixation of the unstable segment, the casualty still shows signs, such as blueness or distressed breathing, of being unable to shift air in and out of the lungs, then it will be necessary to give assisted breathing or artificial respiration.

If you think that a number of ribs are fractured, or that *bleeding is occurring into the chest or lung*—recognized by pain on movement, by frothy spit which is blood-stained and by a rising pulse rate and other signs of internal bleeding—then the casualty, if he is conscious, should be placed in a half-sitting position and inclined towards the injured side. This will allow any blood which collects to sink or flow down to the bottom of the chest cavity on that side *(see Figure 3.18,* page 100). In this position the casualty will breathe most easily because

(a) breathing is easier in a half-sitting position and

(b) less lung compression will result from blood which gravitates to the bottom of the chest cavity.

103

If the casualty is unconscious, he should be placed on the injured side with a slight head-down tip. This allows the good side to function to best advantage and follows the general rules for the treatment of unconsciousness.

REMOVE THE CASUALTY SPEEDILY TO HOSPITAL

In any serious chest injury, as with any other serious injury, arrival of the casualty in hospital should not be delayed any longer than is absolutely necessary in order to carry out any essential treatment which will benefit the casualty. At all times, special efforts should be directed to keeping the airway clear, by encouraging the casualty to cough and to spit out fluid, and in the unconscious casualty by a slight head-down tip and the use of a sucker, if available, to clear accumulated secretions. Breathing should be carefully watched and the colour of the lips, ears and skin should be noted. Obstructed breathing should not occur at this stage if all the right things have been done but nevertheless it should be looked for and treated at once should it occur.

TRANSPORTING CHEST INJURIES

The positions for transporting chest injuries *(Figures 3.21 and 3.22)* are as follows

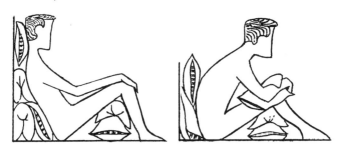

Figure 3.21.—Sitting positions for conscious casualties with chest injuries. Incline to the injured side

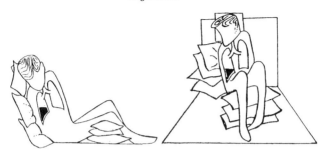

Figure 3.22.—Half-sitting position for conscious casualties with chest injuries

Conscious

Injury to one side.—The casualty should be allowed to take up the position in which he breathes most easily. This will generally be half sitting up and inclined towards the injured side. An alternative position may be leaning forward with the elbows resting on two or three pillows on the thighs or with the forearms resting on a small table.

Injury to both sides.—The best position will probably be half sitting up and inclined towards the worst injured side or leaning forward with the elbows on the knees, as above.

Unconscious

Injury to one side.—The casualty should be placed on the *injured side (Figure 3.23)* in the unconscious position with a slight head-down tip.

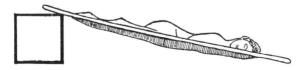

Figure 3.23.—Lay the casualty on the injured side

Injury to both sides.—Place the casualty in the unconscious position on the *worst injured side* with a slight head-down tip. If there is a delay of over an hour in getting to hospital, the casualty should be placed on alternate sides—for about an hour on each side—unless the general condition shows that the casualty breathes much more easily when lying on one side than on the other. If this happens, the casualty should be kept lying on the side which results in the easier breathing.

A NOTE ABOUT THE USE OF SUCKERS AND ANALGESICS IN CHEST INJURIES

There is no doubt that the use of
a sucker
to secure a clear airway can be of tremendous help in any casualty with a serious chest injury. This piece of equipment is essential and should be much more widely available and used. For details of the use of suckers, *see* page 22.

Analgesics (pain relieving drugs) such as morphine and pethidine which depress respiration should not be used for the relief of pain in casualties who have chest injuries (*see* pages 137–142.

THE USE OF OXYGEN IN CHEST INJURIES

There is no doubt that some chest injury casualties will benefit from the administration of oxygen,
but before attempting to give oxygen, it is essential that the casualty has
—a free airway
—adequate breathing movements.
These two conditions should be maintained as far as possible both before and during oxygen administration. *Figure 3.24* shows the causes of difficult or obstructed breathing. For full details of the use of oxygen in first-aid see page 21.

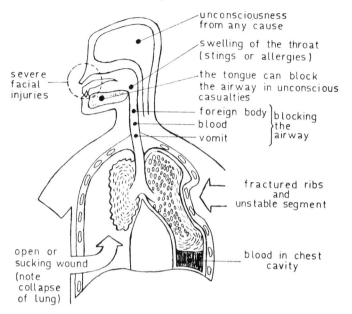

Figure 3.24.—The causes of difficult or obstructed breathing

unconsciousness from any cause

swelling of the throat (stings or allergies)

the tongue can block the airway in unconscious casualties

foreign body }
blood } blocking the airway
vomit }

severe facial injuries

fractured ribs and unstable segment

open or sucking wound (note collapse of lung)

blood in chest cavity

HEART INJURIES

Injuries liable to damage the heart will probably affect the left side of the chest and are likely to be stab and puncture wounds, or crush injuries.

In the case of damage to the heart, there is little that the first-aider can do except to recognize that not much that is effective can be done outside of hospital. So, the problem is to get the casualty speedily to hospital in the best possible condition (*see below*).

A SYNOPSIS OF FIRST-AID for CHEST INJURIES

(*i*) Make sure that the *airway is clear*.
—remove dentures, debris, loose teeth. Mop or suck out blood or vomit in the mouth.
—put head *fully* back with mouth shut in teeth clenched position.
—Suck out again as required to remove any blood, vomit or secretion.

(*ii*) Make sure that *normal breathing movements* can take place.
—Use posture to best advantage.
—Stabilize flail segments.
—Give assisted breathing.
—Give artificial respiration.

(*iii*) Give *oxygen*.

(*iv*) Get the casualty *to hospital*.

ABDOMINAL INJURIES

The surface markings and areas of vulnerability of the various organs are shown in *Figure 3.25*.

Blunt injuries to the abdomen or loin may result in serious internal bleeding from the liver, spleen or kidney. Such injuries may be caused, for example, by an accidental kick in football or by a blunt object in a car smash. The result of a blunt injury may be to crush or split underlying organs, which then bleed. Bleeding can at times be very severe and threatening to life following such blunt injuries. The treatment is that for any internal bleeding. Send the casualty quickly but gently to hospital for blood replacement. He may perhaps need operative treatment to stop the bleeding. Always remember to write down the pulse rate and the time, and some notes about the condition of the casualty. This may help the doctors in hospital.

Blunt injuries to the lowest part of the abdomen may result in a fractured pelvis. The possibility of injury to the

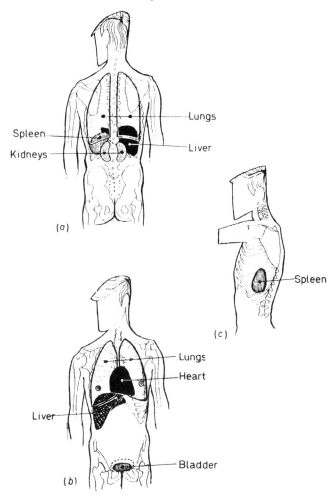

Figure 3.25.—Areas of vulnerability: (a) back, (b) front, (c) left side

bladder or urethra should always be borne in mind when dealing with a fractured pelvis. The casualty should be told not to pass water in case urine escapes into the tissues of the body.

Skin imprinting

Cellular underwear or string vests may leave imprint markings in the skin bruise which follows a blow. This useful, but little known sign, may be of help in assessing the degree of violence in blunt injuries. Where the blow and imprint mark is on skin over a hard area such as ribs, or other underlying bone, the sign is of no value diagnostically—any blow will probably leave a mark.

Where, however, the underlying tissues are soft, as for example over the front of the abdomen, any 'tattooing' will indicate a blunt injury of some severity because the compression force will need to be large in order to leave an imprint. If an imprint is found over any soft area, underlying damage should always be strongly suspected.

WOUNDS OF THE ABDOMEN

Wounds which are on or near the abdomen may communicate with the abdominal cavity. This possibility should always be borne in mind when assessing the severity of any wound in the *lower chest, buttock, groin or crutch areas.*

Puncture wounds, including stab wounds

Puncture wounds may be caused by knives, knitting needles or other sharp objects. Wounds which are *apparently* trivial when viewed from the outside may cause serious damage and bleeding inside. The possibilities of severe bleeding and damage to internal organs such as the liver or bowel make the effects of stab wounds very dangerous indeed.

Therefore, all casualties with stab wounds of the abdomen, chest, buttock and groin should be sent to hospital *at once*, after covering the wound with a sterile dressing.

Abdominal wounds with protrusion of gut

In cases of abdominal wounds with protrusion of gut, cover the gut (bowel) with a clean *damp* cloth, using warm water if possible. Make no attempt to replace any protruded gut. Send the casualty to hospital lying on his back with his knees drawn up—place two or three pillows under the thighs and knees—and with the head forward and supported from behind by two or three pillows or a rolled-up coat.

GENTLE HANDLING AND EARLY SURGERY

Abdominal injuries require very gentle handling to prevent them from becoming worse. In most cases, the successful outcome of the treatment of abdominal wounds and bleeding depends on early surgery, with the additional need in some cases for blood replacement. Such casualties, therefore, should arrive in hospital at the soonest possible time consistent with good first-aid, gentle handling and a comfortable journey to hospital.

EYE INJURIES

PREVENTION

Most eye injuries—and especially those which occur at work—can be prevented by the wearing of suitable eye protection. It is the duty of everyone to help to prevent injuries. Those who treat injuries have a splendid opportunity to point out the lessons of prevention. A minor injury can often be a warning which, if heeded, may prevent serious injuries.

A recent record of eye injuries which occurred in one industry showed that 75 per cent of these injuries were preventable simply by the wearing of suitable eye protection. Five years later the *total* number of eye injuries had fallen to 13 per cent of the previous level, mainly due to considerable efforts to prevent eye injuries by the wearing of

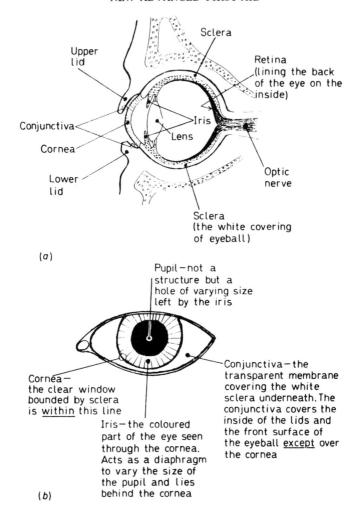

Figure 3.26.—Diagram of the eye: (a) side view, (b) front view

eye protection. However, the percentage of eye injuries out of this lower number which was preventable by wearing eye protection was still high—66 per cent.

MEDICAL INFORMATION

The side and front views of the eye are shown in *Figure 3.26*.

The forms of eye injuries which will frequently present as first-aid problems are:

—injuries to the eyelids;

—foreign bodies (for example, grit, dust, dirt, metallic particles)

    loose under the lids or on the eyeball,

    stuck (embedded) in the surface of the eyball or

    inside the eyeball (intraocular foreign bodies);

—injuries to the eyeball caused by

    sharp objects (for example, knives, needles, fish hooks) or

    blunt objects (for example, fists, cricket balls, snowballs);

—burns

    heat (for example, a cigarette burn, or a hot foreign body as in metal work),

    chemical (for example, caustic soda splashes) or

    ultraviolet ('arc eyes', or 'welder's flash', 'snow blindness').

INJURIES TO THE EYELIDS

If the eyeball is undamaged, the treatment of injuries to the eyelids will follow the general line of wound treatment—stop bleeding, prevent infection and send the casualty to hospital. A pad and bandage to cover the lids will usually be the appropriate and comforting treatment.

If the eyelids are torn or displaced, they should be carefully repositioned before applying the pad and bandage. A pad and bandage should *not* be applied directly to the eyeball. If the injury is such that the lids do not cover the eyeball, build up a dressing around the eyeball and bandage over this dressing before sending the casualty to hospital.

FOREIGN BODIES

Loose foreign bodies should be removed by means of a moistened wool-tipped applicator. A foreign body which is thought to be loose but which does not come off the surface of the eye with one gentle wipe should be treated as if it was stuck. *No further attempts should be made by the first-aider to remove the foreign body.*

Foreign bodies which are stuck to the surface of the eye should not be removed by a first-aider. Stuck foreign bodies should be treated by covering the eye with a pad and bandage, and sending the casualty to hospital.

Foreign bodies which are thought to be partly *inside* the eyeball should be treated by covering the eye with a pad and bandage. Particular care should be taken to build dressings up around large stuck foreign bodies and eyelid tears in order to keep the dressing off the eyeball itself and to prevent the dressing applying pressure to the foreign body

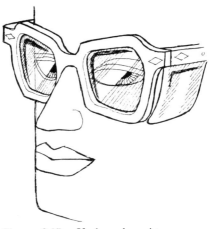

Figure 3.27.—If hazards exist, wear eye protection

and perhaps, therefore, increasing the amount of eye damage.

High-speed fragments

Sometimes very small fragments of metal or some other hard material will enter the inside of the eye due to the high speed at which they are travelling when they hit the eye. Such fragments are then referred to as intraocular foreign bodies. The casualty may feel impact or pain at the time such foreign bodies enter the eye, *OR he may feel little or NOTHING.* Such injuries occur most often after striking a steel chisel or punch with a hammer. Drilling, milling, grinding, boring, hammering or chipping may give rise to high-speed fragments which can become stuck or embedded in the surface of the eyeball or which can actually penetrate and enter the inside of the eyeball.

Eye protection must ALWAYS be worn when doing these jobs *(Figure 3.27)*.

Never use, or allow others to use, a 'mushroomed' chisel. Many eyes are lost each year due to metallic fragments flying off the mushroomed head of the chisel and severely damaging the eye.

If a casualty thinks that he may have been struck in the eye or if he has a painful eye subsequent to doing any job which gives rise to high-speed fragments, *then he MUST be sent to hospital to see a doctor even if there is no visible wound, tear or abnormality of the eyeball or eyelids.*

If you know of a special eye department or eye hospital near, this is the ideal place to send the casualty.

Occasionally, high-speed fragments give rise to bleeding under the conjunctiva—a subjunctival haemorrhage. The conjunctiva is the fine transparent membrane which covers the white of the eyeball and the inside of the eyelids. This bleeding can be seen as a bright red patch on the white part of the eyeball. Such casualties must always be seen by a doctor.

SHARP INJURIES TO THE EYE

Wounds of the eyeball should be treated by covering the eye with a pad and bandage and sending the casualty to hospital.

BLUNT INJURIES TO THE EYE

The small hard rubber balls used for squash and racketball are particularly dangerous in causing eyeball compression injuries. If the eyeball is squeezed or compressed by a blow from any blunt object, the inner lining of the eyeball may be damaged and may subsequently detach from the

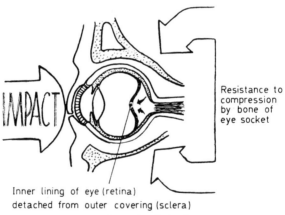

IMPACT

Resistance to compression by bone of eye socket

Inner lining of eye (retina) detached from outer covering (sclera)

Figure 3.28.—How a detached retina can occur

outer covering (a detached retina) *(Figure 3.28)*. When this happens, vision is lost over the area which is detached. If the small central black area is detached (the area which deals with most vision except that which is described as seen 'out of the corner of the eye') the loss of vision can be severely disabling. Fortunately, if the condition is diagnosed immediately, the inner lining can usually be 'spot welded' back into place. An opacity of the lens of the eye (a cataract) may be a late result of a blunt injury.

Therefore, any

—black eye, or

—blunt injury to the eye, which gives rise to any actual or suspected loss of vision or to any bleeding or redness of the eye,

should be sent to hospital to be seen by a doctor.

If there is no wound of the eye there is no need to cover the eye unless bright light hurts it.

BURNS OF THE EYE

Heat burns

If there is a heat burn of the eyelids or of the eyeball, this should be cooled by water in the usual way (page 159). If after the removal of a small loose foreign body, a burn of the eyeball is found, close the eyelids and apply a pad and bandage. The casualty should be sent to hospital for further treatment.

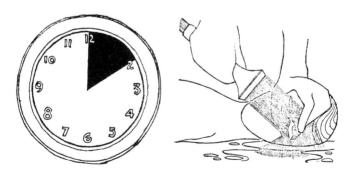

Figure 3.29.—Hold the eyelids apart and wash for 10 minutes

Chemical burns

Wash the eye(s) IMMEDIATELY to remove and flush out the chemical. Use the nearest source of water—from a tap, shower, hose or jug. Act immediately to get the chemical flushed out of the eye.

(a) Turn the head towards the affected side to prevent the chemical flowing into, and injuring, the other eye.

(b) Irrigate the eye(s) with copious amounts of tap water. Separate the eyelids with your fingers so that the water can wash the chemical away from the inside of lids and from the eyeball. Continue for 10 minutes timed *by the clock (Figure 3.29). DO NOT SKIMP OR HURRY THIS STEP.*

(c) Gently cover the closed eye(s) with a sterile pad and bandage.

(d) Send the casualty to hospital as soon as possible.

Alkali burns tend to be more damaging to the eye than acid burns. This is because acids can be washed out more easily. Alkalis tend to combine chemically with the surface layers of the eyelids and eyeball (they bind to the protein) and are thus less easy to wash out. The alkali is then slowly released from the surface layers when these layers are damaged by the chemical, and it can then cause further chemical burning and damage.

The moral of all this may be listed as follows.

(i) Avoid chemical burns of the eye. They are preventable by appropriate precautions. Try to encourage everyone to adopt sound preventive attitudes. Loss of vision is very high price to pay for neglect of safe work methods.

(ii) If chemical injuries do occur, wash the eye out *immediately*, and continue washing for 10 minutes timed by the clock. Do not skimp or hurry this step of washing out the eye with large amounts of water.

(iii) Remember that alkali burns are especially damaging and give such casualties *prolonged* irrigation—say, 20 minutes timed by the clock.

Lime burns.—In the case of lime burns (alkali), after an initial good irrigation, look quickly for, and remove, any obvious solid particles. Then, irrigate again for at least 10 minutes timed by the clock before repeating the whole process. Finally, cover the eye(s) and send the casualty to hospital.

Ultraviolet burns ('arc eye' or 'welder's flash', 'snow blindness')

The casualty, who has usually been near an electric welding arc or otherwise exposed to ultraviolet radiation, has a sensation of grittiness or sandiness, accompanied in more severe cases by pain and dislike of bright light. The symptoms often develop late at night or early in the morning, because the effects of an ultraviolet burn are not immediately felt. Both eyes will usually be uniformly pink or red over the areas which are normally exposed with the eyes open—but not elsewhere. Always look for foreign bodies in case they are also present.

Treat an ultraviolet burn of the eyes by bathing the eyes with ice cold water, or the coldest obtainable. Dark glasses or darkness and two soluble (buffered) aspirin tablets will give relief in mild cases. More severe cases with painful watery eyes and much dislike of light should be sent, wearing dark glasses or pads and bandages, to hospital or to a doctor.

CAUTION

Ultraviolet burns almost always affect BOTH eyes. The one-eyed 'flash' is usually due to an embedded foreign body. NEVER treat one red eye as a 'flash'—send such a casualty to hospital with a pad and bandage over the red eye.

Protection against ultraviolet light. When there is any danger of the eyes being exposed to high levels of ultraviolet light, for example, in electric welding, in the use of sun lamps or in snow-fields even in overcast conditions, always wear suitable eye protection. For snow, dark glasses offer ample protection.

Burns of the retina. NEVER look directly at the sun or at an eclipse. Severe and permanently disabling injury to the eyes can be caused by looking at the sun or at eclipses through a telescope or binoculars. Dark glasses—even several pairs— do not offer protection against serious burning to the back of the eye (the retina) if people look at the sun directly.

The correct way to observe an eclipse at home is to make a pinhole in a piece of paper and allow the sun to shine through this and onto another larger sheet. The sun and eclipse shadows can then be observed *indirectly*.

FRACTURES

MEDICAL INFORMATION

A fracture is a break or crack in a bone. There are three main ways in which a bone can be broken.

(*i*) *Direct violence*
A kick on the shin which breaks the bone at the site of the blow is a good example of a fracture by direct violence.

(*ii*) *Indirect violence*
In the case of indirect violence, the fracture occurs away from the site of impact or force. An example is a fracture of the lower part of the spine due to landing on the feet after jumping 5 metres (16 feet). The impact is transmitted through the bones of the legs and the pelvis to the spine. A spiral fracture of the leg bones due to trapping of the foot and a rotation of the body is another example of indirect violence. Other fractures due to indirect violence are found at the neck of the femur and the collar bone (clavicle).

(*iii*) *Muscular action*
In some places, the pull of muscles can be enough to cause fractures. Examples of this are a fracture of the knee-

cap due to the pull of strong thigh muscles, and a fracture of the ribs due to violent muscular action in coughing.

Fractures can be classified as closed or open. A *closed* fracture has *no* wound at or near it, while an *open* fracture has a wound at or near it leading to the site of the fracture.

Fractures can usually be *diagnosed* by the history of injury, and by pain, tenderness, deformity, swelling, loss of use and unnatural movement. In first-aid, suspected fractures must always be treated as fractures.

The AIMS of FIRST-AID for FRACTURES

Firstly, cover all open fractures to prevent infection and to stop bleeding; secondly, prevent further damage and reduce pain by preventing movement occurring round the break—that is, immobilize the fracture; and lastly, send the casualty to hospital for further treatment.

We do not intend here to repeat the details of the first-aid treatment of fractures but shall comment only on a few points which are additional to, or which clarify, the information already given in *New Essential First Aid*.

ESTIMATING BLOOD LOSS ASSOCIATED WITH FRACTURES

In advanced first-aid, a more accurate assessment can be made of the severity of injuries, of the need for blood replacement—and thus of individual priorities—by estimating the likely blood loss from each fracture or other injury.

INFLATABLE SPLINTS

Fractures are an important cause of blood loss, usually by internal bleeding. Reference should be made again to *Figure 2.2* which gives details of blood losses by injuries.

Experience in using inflatable splints has shown that they are probably the most suitable and easily applied form of immobilization for *below*-elbow and *below*-knee fractures. The splints are NOT suitable for other fractures. In order to prevent over-inflation and the possible circulatory trouble resulting from it, the splints should be inflated by mouth and not with a pump. With this proviso, inflatable splints provide support, and x-rays in hospital can be taken without removing the splint. However, they are expensive and easily damaged.

PLASTER OF PARIS EMERGENCY SPLINTING

> '*In first aid, fractures of the limbs should be made comfortable and, if necessary, splinted.*'
> P. S. LONDON, FRCS

London's aphorism is very apt, and when splinting is necessary, there may be a few occasions where a rigid but moulded splint such as can be made from plaster of Paris will be best.

The use of plaster of Paris slabs as a means of immobilizing fractures or suspected fractures or fracture-dislocations is particularly useful if a casualty has a long and perhaps difficult journey to face before he can have definitive treatment. For example, a broken arm or ankle sustained on a mountain may mean a long and arduous journey for the casualty over rocky terrain. Plaster of Paris splinting under such conditions can add much to the comfort and safety of the casualty and helps to prevent complications.

Plaster of Paris bandages, which are bandages impregnated with plaster of Paris, are made folded on top of each other in lengths to make a five-thickness slab of appropriate length. After wetting, the slab is moulded to the limb and bandaged on. The plaster of Paris will set sufficiently within about 5–10 minutes to produce a firm support for the injured part, and will grow stronger as it dries. Suitable kits are available consisting of two plaster slabs, 5 ply, 15 cm ×

76 cm (6 × 30 inches), and two bandages contained in a polythene bag. When the kit has to be used, the bag is opened without removing the contents and is then filled with water to within 5 cm (2 inches) of the top. Use tepid water if possible; this is comfortable for the casualty and leads to a convenient rate of setting in the plaster of Paris. The first slab is removed, squeezed to remove excess water and is then ready for application. The kit is 15 cm × 15 cm × 5 cm (6 × 6 × 2 inches) in size, and weighs 710 g (22 oz). Instructions are included with every kit.

Before discussing details of application, five general points must be considered in connection with plaster of Paris splints—safety, strength, moulding, length and recording of information on the plaster.

Safety

There must always be a part of the circumference of the limb left free of the plaster of Paris splint (Figure 3.30). Emergency

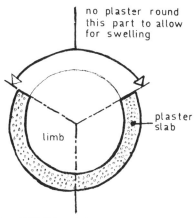

no plaster round
this part to allow
for swelling

plaster
slab

limb

Figure 3.30.—NEVER encircle more than two-thirds of the circumference of the limb. ALWAYS leave room for swelling

splinting must NEVER encircle the limb completely. This is because swelling occurs round most injuries, and if this swelling grows and is tightly contained, the swelling may cut off the blood supply to the limb at and below the swelling. Absence of blood supply may mean severe damage to the limb or even complete loss.

Strength

After application the splint must always be bandaged on to the limb—an unsupported slab breaks easily. Splints should also be moulded *not more than* two-thirds round the limb. The curved section adds to the strength and helps to keep the splint in place. Five thicknesses of bandage folded on top of each other to make a five-thickness slab will be suitable for women and children. Men probably need a seven-thickness slab.

Moulding

When the plaster of Paris is applied to the limb, it must be free of wrinkles and bumps on the inside, and must be carefully moulded to conform to the contours of the limb. Any wrinkles or lumps in the slab will become hard edges or sticking out points when the plaster sets. Use only the flat of the palm or the flat of the fingers when moulding a plaster. DO NOT dent the plaster with your finger tips—this will lead to real discomfort. Even support will not be given if the slab is unevenly applied. Take special care not to make creases at joint folds such as behind the knee and in front of the ankle. Any unduly prominent contour, for example, the ankles in thin casualties, may require a little padding, using some cotton wool or other soft substance, over the prominence before the plaster slab is applied in order to prevent pressure. No encircling bandages should ever be used under a plaster to hold padding or wound dressings in place. Use sticky tape in small pieces or nothing at all.

Length

To secure adequate immobilization, sufficient and appropriate length of splinting must be applied. Make sure that the edges of the plaster slabs are well clear of the bends of joints, for example, the elbow, and if possible leave the fingers clear.

Information on the plaster

Always write the time of application clearly on the outside of the plaster. It is often helpful, too, to illustrate the injuries diagrammatically on the outside of the plaster for the benefit of all who may attend the casualty *en route* to hospital.

APPLYING PLASTER OF PARIS SPLINTS

Plaster slabs may be applied over wound dressing or over thin articles of clothing such as socks, but not over any thick article. Remove rings and jewellery so that constriction due to swelling is prevented. *Never* apply encircling turns of bandage under a plaster.

SPLINT FOR ANKLE AND FOOT INJURIES (BELOW-KNEE SPLINT)

Use a below-knee splint for fractures or suspected fractures to the ankle and foot which are in the shaded areas of

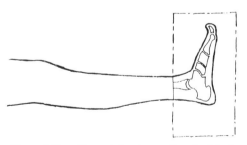

Figure 3.31.—Use a below-knee splint for injuries here

125

Figure 3.31. Do not use this splint for any fracture above the ankle—an above-knee plaster is required for shin bone and knee injuries.

This splint may conveniently be applied with the casualty lying face down and with the knee bent *(Figure 3.32)*

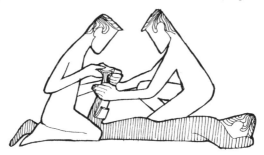

Figure 3.32.—Applying a below-knee plaster splint in face-down position to a stable fracture

if the fracture is stable, that is, does not move or slide on itself. If, however, the fracture is unstable, and moves, the splint should be applied while the casualty is lying on his back and with an assistant steadying and applying traction to the foot *(Figure 3.33)*. The foot should be kept at right

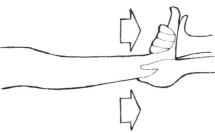

Figure 3.33.—Use traction when applying a plaster splint to unstable fractures

angles to the leg. Make sure that the traction is continuous and not intermittent.

Method (Figure 3.34)

(*i*) Apply a back slab from behind the knee to the base of the toes. Do not go beyond the base of the toes. Fold back any excess to make sure the area of the skin at the back of the knee is quite free from plaster.

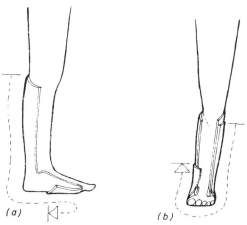

Figure 3.34.—A below-knee splint. (a) Apply a back slab to the base of the toes and turn over (and down) any excess. (b) Apply a second slab over the first, beginning at the outside, and wrap it round the instep and up the inside of the leg

(*ii*) Apply the second slab to the outer side of the leg starting in line with and on top of the first slab, to leave the front of the skin clear. Bring the second slab round over the sole of the foot and then as far up the inner side of the leg as it will go.

(*iii*) Fix the slabs to the leg, using the bandages. In the case of an unstable fracture, apply the back slab as above.

Maintain traction on the foot and keep it at a right angle to the leg until the back slab dries and solidifies somewhat. Then apply the U slab and so on.

SPLINT FOR LEG AND KNEE INJURIES (FULL-LEG SPLINT)

Use a full-leg splint for fractures or suspected fractures from above the ankle to just above the knee (*Figure 3.35*).

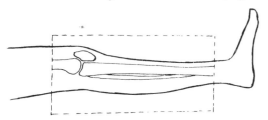

Figure 3.35.—Use a full-leg splint for injuries here

This includes injuries to the shin bone (tibia), to the knee joint and to the lower end of the thigh bone (femur). Mid-thigh injuries and above will not benefit from an above-knee plaster as not enough immobilization will be provided.

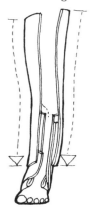

Figure 3.36—A full-leg splint. Make a below-knee plaster and add two slabs on the sides, the inner one beginning in the crutch

Method

Two packs (four slabs) are required.

(*i*) Make a below-knee splint (as shown in *Figure 3.34*).

(*ii*) Apply two further slabs to the outside and to the inside of the lower limb *(Figure 3.36)*. The inside slab should begin as high up the thigh as it will comfortably go in the crutch. The outside slab should begin slightly higher than the inner one, over the most prominent part of the outside of the leg. This prominence is the upper end of the thigh bone (femur) just below hip joint level.

(*iii*) Apply the crêpe paper bandages to fix the slabs.

SPLINT FOR WRIST AND HAND INJURIES (FOREARM SPLINT)

Use a forearm splint for fractures or suspected fractures of the wrist and below and for fractures of the *lower end* of the forearm bones *(Figure 3.37(a))*.

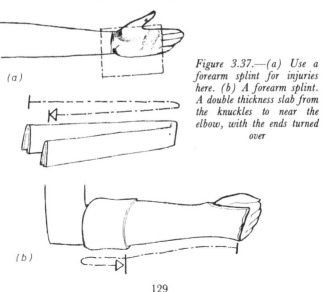

(*a*)

(*b*)

Figure 3.37.—(a) Use a forearm splint for injuries here. (b) A forearm splint. A double thickness slab from the knuckles to near the elbow, with the ends turned over

Method (Figure 3.37(b))

Only one slab is required.

(*i*) Double the slab lengthways.

(*ii*) Apply the double-thickness slab from the knuckles at the base of the fingers to just below the elbow. Fold over both ends. This makes a rounded edge.

(*iii*) Bandage the slab in place with a bandage, taking turns round the wrist and across the palm of the hand between the thumb and index finger.

SPLINT FOR FOREARM AND ELBOW INJURIES (FULL-ARM SPLINT)

Use a full-arm splint for fractures or suspected fractures from above the wrist up to and including the elbow (*Figure 3.38*).

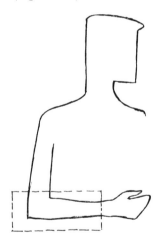

Figure 3.38.—Use a full-arm splint for injuries here

Method

One pack (two slabs) is required.

(*i*) Apply one slab from the knuckles at the base of the fingers along the back of the arm and forearm (*Figure 3.39(a)*)

130

and thence round the elbow and back down the inner side of the forearm as far as it will reach. Keep the elbow at a right angle or nearly so.

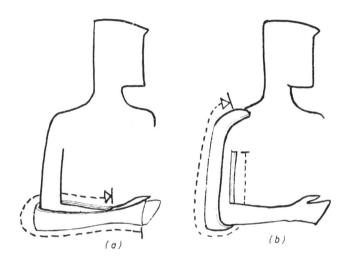

Figure 3.39.—A full-arm splint. (a) First, apply a slab from the knuckles up the forearm, round the elbow and down the inside of the forearm. (b) Then apply a second slab from the arm-pit down the inner side of the arm, round the elbow and up the outside of the arm to the shoulder. Keep front of elbow clear of slabs and bandages

(*ii*) Apply the second slab, beginning in the arm-pit, downwards along the inner side of the arm and thence round the elbow and up the outer side of the arm and over the shoulder as far as it will go.

MAKE SURE THAT THE SLABS DO NOT OVER-LAP AT THE FRONT OF THE ELBOW. TURN THE SLABS BACK SO AS TO LEAVE PLENTY OF ROOM FOR SWELLING AT THIS SITE.

(*iii*) Bandage the slabs on with the crêpe paper bandages. *Do not bandage over the front of the elbow.*

(*iv*) Keep the arm into the side of the body while the plaster sets. Apply a suitable sling (broad sling or collar-and-cuff) when the plaster has set.

SPLINT FOR ARM INJURIES (UPPER-ARM SPLINT)

The upper-arm splint is used for any fracture or suspected fracture above the elbow *(Figure 3.40(a))*. Only one slab is required.

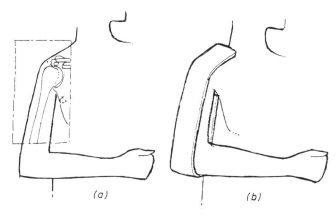

Figure 3.40.—(a) Use an upper-arm splint for injuries here. (b) An upper-arm splint, beginning at the top of the shoulder, down the outside of the arm, round the elbow and up the inside of the arm

Method

(*i*) Apply the slab to the outer side of the arm and shoulder, beginning at the shoulder tip *(Figure 3.40(b))*. Continue the slab round the elbow and as far up the inner side of the arm as it will go.

(*ii*) Bandage, taking care not to bandage over the front of the elbow.

(*iii*) Apply a collar-and-cuff sling.

DANGER TO CIRCULATION

Remember to check the circulation of blood to the fingers or toes when you have applied the splints and bandages. Swelling may make the splint tight and tend to obstruct the blood flow. The appearance of fingers and toes is summarized in Table 3.2.

TABLE 3.2

Normal	Danger signs
Pink	White, purple or blue
Warm	Cold to the touch, not necessarily cold to the casualty
Light touch felt easily	Altered sensation or numbness

When swelling occurs, check *frequently* to make sure that no danger signs of circulatory obstruction occur. If any of the danger signs appear, loosen the bandages and remove the slabs until normal circulation is restored. Then, refix or remake the slabs in such a way that the danger will not recur.

OPEN FRACTURES OR WOUNDS—A CAUTIONARY NOTE
ABOUT FIXING WOUND DRESSINGS

If wounds are present, the wounds should be covered by dressings. The dressings should, if required, be lightly fixed using sticky tape. The plaster slab(s) are then moulded directly over the dressings. Wound dressings should NOT be bandaged in place by encircling turns of roller bandages and then covered by plaster slabs, in case the circulation to the limb is impaired.

CRUSH INJURIES

TRAPPED CASUALTIES

Crush injuries often mean a trapped casualty. Unless the casualty is in immediate danger from his environment or from other injuries, the crushed and trapped casualty should be freed according to a carefully worked out plan. Adequate help should be sought and available before tackling the job of releasing the casualty. Fire brigades are usually equipped to deal with wreckage and if the police and/or ambulance authorities are informed of the problem of crushing and trapping, they will send suitable help. It may also be wise to *send at once for medical assistance*, particularly if the casualty is going to be some time in being released, if the amount of trapping is large or if there is suspicion of damage to any vital organ.

Two forms of crush injuries can be distinguished:
—crush injuries which involve vital organs such as brain, lungs or liver, and
—crush injuries of limbs.

CRUSH INJURIES WHICH INVOLVE VITAL ORGANS

The treatment of crush injuries which involve vital organs will, after release of trapping, follow the same lines as the treatment of damage to the brain, lung or liver from any cause. These problems have been dealt with earlier in the various sections on head, chest and abdominal injuries.

CRUSH INJURIES OF LIMBS

An injury which traps one hand will not give rise to serious *general* effects when the casualty is released. On the other hand, an injury which traps a leg from the upper thigh to the foot may—and probably will—give rise to serious general effects. As a rough guide, the severity of the general effects of crushing in limb injuries will be proportional to the amount of tissue which is crushed and damaged.

INJURIES

Following release of crushed limbs, the blood vessels in the crushed and damaged areas will be unable to retain fluid. Plasma and/or blood will leak into the tissues of the crushed area. In this way, quite large quantities of fluid and/or blood may be lost to the circulation. This will soon give rise to general effects.

The AIMS of FIRST-AID for CRUSH INJURIES of LIMBS

(1) Release from trapping.
(2) Prevent bleeding.
(3) Prevent infection.
(4) Prevent further damage to the limb.
(5) Send the casualty to hospital.

RELEASE FROM TRAPPING

Make sure that in releasing the casualty he will not suffer further injury by pulling, tugging or by further falls of material. Protect the casualty from any jagged edges and handle him gently.

PREVENT BLEEDING

Follow the usual pattern of pressing where the blood comes from—preferably with a sterile dressing—and, if injuries permit, elevating the arm or leg.

PREVENT INFECTION

Wounds should be dressed in the usual way with a sterile dressing. Crushed limbs tend to swell a lot when circulation of blood is restored due to leakage of blood and plasma out of the damaged blood vessels. It is therefore wise to use crêpe or conforming bandages which can stretch to bandage dressings in place. Care should be taken not to impair circulation by tight or constrictive bandaging.

PREVENT FURTHER DAMAGE TO THE LIMB

Fractures or suspected fractures should be immobilized.

SEND THE CASUALTY TO HOSPITAL

If the amount of tissue crushed has been large—say from mid-thigh downwards in both legs—the amount of plasma and blood loss could be life-threatening (*see* blood loss by injuries, page 43, and fluid loss, page 33). Such casualties need to reach hospital soon for plasma and/or blood replacement.

If the crushing has been large in amount and the journey to hospital will take more than $1-1\frac{1}{2}$ hours an intravenous plasma or plasma-expander infusion will help to combat the fluid loss from the circulation until the casualty reaches hospital. The time to start the infusion is just before or immediately after release. It is for this amongst other reasons that medical help should be sought at an early stage. There is no place for fluids by mouth in first-aid for crush injuries.

Watch carefully for any constriction which may develop due to bandages or splintage being involved with swelling. Check that no tight bands develop. Do not place heavy blankets over crushed limbs—use a cage to keep the weight of the blankets off the limb (*see Figure 4.7*, page 176).

The circulation in crushed limbs may be very poor so be especially careful that you do not make it worse by bad treatment. Note especially the temperature and colour of the fingers or toes after release. They may not resume normal colour. It is important to observe that they do not become worse following release from trapping because a constriction is produced or allowed to develop.

See also the remarks on pages 19–28 about circulatory stagnation and the use of oxygen in crush injuries.

THE CONTROL OF PAIN IN FIRST-AID

In first-aid the control of pain can be discussed under two main headings.

(1) The control of pain *without* drugs
>Gentle handling.
>Stop movement of injured parts.
>Transport carefully.
>Reassurance and relief of anxiety.

(2) The control of pain *with* drugs
>Minor pain.
>Severe pain.

(1) CONTROL OF PAIN WITHOUT DRUGS

Much pain can be *avoided* by gentle handling, by the omission of panic handling, by stopping movement of injured parts, by elevation of limbs and by careful transport of the casualty. There is no place for panic handling in good first-aid. Speed in scooping a casualty onto a stretcher and getting him behind the closed doors of an ambulance does not necessarily correlate with efficient or good first-aid. If rough handling is involved, it is certainly bad first-aid.

The effect of existing pain can be mitigated by relieving the natural anxiety of any casualty who is in pain. A confident, gentle and reassuring manner in dealing with the injuries will always produce a lessening of anxiety and tension in the casualty, when pain may be felt to be less severe.

(2) CONTROL OF PAIN WITH DRUGS

Minor pain

In attempting to control minor pain by drugs as a first-aid measure, we assume that minor pain arises from injuries which are in themselves not serious—for example, a single fracture of a limb or a painful bruise.

The general rule that injured casualties, except burned casualties, some poisoned casualties, or the victims of chilling by immersion or wet–cold exposure, should be given nothing by mouth, should only be broken by an experienced advanced first-aider if

- (*i*) it is CERTAIN that the casualty will NOT require an ANAESTHETIC on arrival in hospital, and
- (*ii*) there is other good reason for wishing to break the by-mouth rule. Good reasons might include complaints of pain from the casualty after the condition has been treated as far as possible by gentle handling and reassurance. Good reasons may also include a journey over rough ground and delay in reaching hospital. Under such circumstances, the advanced first-aider may consider the giving of simple pain-relieving drugs to the conscious casualty.

Two drugs are useful.

(*a*) *Soluble aspirin tablet* (300 mg).—Soluble aspirin tablets may be given to an adult in a dose of 2 tablets dissolved in or taken with a little water. Children require smaller doses.

Before giving soluble aspirin tablets, always enquire whether the casualty is allergic to aspirin, has any form of indigestion or ulcer trouble, or whether he finds that aspirin upsets his stomach. If the answer to any of these questions is yes, do not give soluble aspirin. Do not give aspirin to children under 2 years of age.

(*b*) *Paracetamol tablet* (500 mg).—Paracetamol tablets may be given to those who cannot be given soluble aspirin tablets for the reasons outlined above. Paracetamol tablets may be given to an adult in a dose of 2 tablets with a little water.

Severe pain

Two drugs can be used for the relief of severe pain in first-aid—pethidine and morphine.

The use of both of these drugs is controlled and they can only be prescribed by a doctor. We also believe, for the reasons given below, that apart from very highly exceptional circumstances these drugs should only be given in first-aid *by a doctor* or that the drug should be administered *under the immediate guidance of a doctor*. Much of what follows will therefore be of interest to the first-aider, but is mainly of concern to doctors.

Both of these drugs can do considerable harm as well as good and, if given in the wrong dosage and/or by the wrong route, may affect the casualty adversely. For example, both are respiratory depressants and should not be given to casualties who have head, chest or abdominal injuries, or suspected injuries to these areas. Pethidine is also capable of reacting adversely with certain tranquillizer drugs (monoamine oxidase inhibitors). It is important to recognize that the *only* indication in first-aid for the use of pethidine or morphine is to relieve *severe* pain. These drugs should NOT be given to badly injured people as a routine. Many badly injured casualties do not suffer pain and therefore do not require to be given pain-relieving drugs.

Pethidine or morphine?—Some believe that as a first-aid measure for relieving pain pethidine is superior to morphine, because in seriously injured casualties enough morphine cannot be given intravenously to provide relief of pain without depressing the casualty's general condition.

Morphine is, however, advocated by many as the preferred drug for the relief of severe pain in first-aid. A comparison of the properties of pethidine and morphine is listed in Table 3.3. Until a clear consensus emerges, the reader will have to make his own choice. The weight of opinion at present seems to be greater on the side of using morphine than pethidine, *provided that the rules which are given later are scrupulously followed*.

Contra-indications.—Pethidine and morphine are both respiratory depressants and in seriously injured casualties can easily give rise to weak breathing or even cause breathing

TABLE 3.3

Pethidine, given intravenously	Morphine sulphate, given intravenously
Effective in mild to moderate pain	Effective in severe pain
Respiratory depressant	Respiratory depressant
Non-euphoric*	Euphoric*
Dangerous with some tranquillizers (monoamine oxidase inhibitors)	No special risk with tranquillizers
When blood volume is low, may cause marked general and respiratory depression	When blood volume is low, may cause marked general and respiratory depression
May cause local inflammation of the vein (phlebitis) unless in dilute solution	No local reaction
Tendency to cause vomiting	Tendency to cause vomiting
Dangerous in asthma sufferers	Dangerous in asthma sufferers

* A drug is said to be euphoric if it produces a considerable elevation of mood. An extreme degree of euphoria could be represented by a seriously injured casualty who was benignly happy and quite unconcerned about his condition.

to stop if given in too large amounts. Do not give pethidine or morphine to people who suffer from asthma.

The presence of head injury or suspected head injury, chest injury or suspected chest injury and abdominal injury or suspected abdominal injury are absolute contra-indications to the use of morphine and pethidine, because these drugs may mask the signs of head and abdominal injuries, and in chest injuries will, by respiratory depressant action, adversely affect the injury.

Casualties who have lost a lot of blood from their circulation (hypovolaemia) are very easily overwhelmed by doses of pethidine or morphine which are tolerated well by normal people. It is probably wise, therefore, to withhold these drugs from such casualties.

Suggested rules for pethidine and morphine administration in first-aid

We would therefore propose the following rules for the administration of pethidine and morphine in first-aid.

(1) The drug should *only be given by a doctor*, or in the presence of a doctor under his direct supervision by another person of adequate training and experience.

    (2a) The drug should *not be given* in the presence of
        a head injury or suspected head injury,
        a chest injury or suspected chest injury,

    (2b) The drug should be given *with extreme care, slowly, and in the smallest amount required to relieve pain* in the presence of
        an abdominal injury or suspected abdominal injury,
        considerable blood loss from the circulation (hypovolaemia).

(3) The *only indication* for these drugs is *severe pain*. The presence of severe injuries is NOT an indication for giving morphine. Nor should pethidine be given in these circumstances. Many casualties who are severely injured do not feel pain—their perception is altered. Such casualties have often suffered also from considerable blood loss from the circulation and from head, chest or abdominal injuries— all of which are contra-indications to the administration of morphine or pethidine.

(4) The drug should be given *intravenously or not at all*.

(5) The casualty should be given the *smallest amount* of the drug which will *relieve pain*. Give half the amount which you estimate may be required and wait before giving more, to see the effect. After a suitable interval, give more if required, again in small amounts followed by a pause. Beware of overdosage, especially if the casualty has lost blood from his circulation.

(6) *A note to the hospital* must always be plainly affixed to, or marked on, the casualty. This note should state the amount of drug given, the route of administration, and the time at

which the drug was given. Neglect of this rule has resulted in overdosage.

Failure to follow these rules, for example, in the use of morphine, has led to unnecessary deaths. If morphine cannot be given intravenously, it is better not to give it at all, because the drug may not be absorbed from a subcutaneous or intra-muscular injection in a casualty who has a failing or deficient peripheral circulation. This may lead to increased dosage in an attempt to relieve pain. When such a casualty is given blood in hospital and the circulation improves, large amounts of morphine are then released from the injection site and cause respiratory and generalized depression which may be fatal.

Giving pethidine intravenously.—A solution of pethidine containing 50 mg of pethidine in 5 ml of distilled water (10 mg to 1 ml) is used.

In adults 10–20 mg of pethidine (1–2 ml of pethidine solution) is slowly given intravenously and the effect is noted. The needle is not withdrawn from the vein until sufficient pethidine has been given to relieve pain. Further small divided doses of 10 mg are given until relief from pain is obtained. The needle is then withdrawn.

Giving morphine intravenously.—A solution of morphine sulphate containing 10 mg in 1 ml of distilled water is used. Approximately half the estimated required dose is injected intravenously. Large adults who have not lost much blood could have a starting dose of 5 mg. Wait for about 30–45 seconds to assess the effect. Further divided doses may then be given until relief from pain is obtained. Finally, the needle is withdrawn.

CHAPTER 4

THE EFFECTS OF HEAT AND COLD

Feare no more the heate o' th' Sun,
Nor the furious Winters rages . . . .
William Shakespeare

In this chapter we shall consider the general and local effects of heat and cold. The general effects of heat give rise to heat illness, while the local effects of heat are burns. The general effect of cold is to cause chilling. We shall discuss chilling in two parts: first, the sudden chilling of fit adults or young people which may occur following immersion in cold water, or on the mountains due to wet–cold exposure; and second, the slower chilling which gives rise to illness in the specially susceptible groups of young babies and old people. The local effect of cold gives rise to frostbite.

Chilling of the body is often referred to as *hypo*thermia and overheating as *hyper*thermia. Chilling may arise suddenly, giving rise to *acute* hypothermia; or it may come on more slowly, resulting in *subacute* or *chronic* hypothermia. Similar use can be made of the terms acute, subacute and chronic in relation to hyperthermia.

We shall therefore discuss the effects of heat and cold as follows.

HEAT
    The GENERAL effects of heat
        heat illness (*salt/fluid depletion*)
        heat illness (*hyperpyrexia*)
    The LOCAL effects of heat
        burns and scalds

COLD
   The GENERAL effects of cold
      acute hypothermia
      immersion chilling
      wet–cold chilling
      subacute or chronic hypothermia
      chilling in babies and old people
   The LOCAL effects of cold
      frostbite

THE GENERAL EFFECTS OF HEAT
MEDICAL INFORMATION

Two forms of heat illness may present as first-aid problems.
      Heat illness (*salt/fluid depletion*)
      Heat illness (*hyperpyrexia*)

Heat illness (salt/fluid depletion) is caused by depletion of salt or fluid in the body. Two forms may be described:
      heat cramps, and
      heat exhaustion

Heat cramps, a mild form of the illness, is characterized by painful muscular contractions, and is due to salt depletion. *Heat exhaustion* is a more severe type of heat illness and is due to a combination of salt and fluid (water) depletion.

Heat illness (hyperpyrexia), also known as 'heat stroke', is characterized by an abnormally raised body temperature.

NORMAL HEAT REGULATION

In order to understand heat illness, it is useful to have some knowledge of the mechanisms of heat production and heat loss from the body, and of normal heat regulation.

Heat production

There is always a background production of heat from the basic body processes such as breathing, heart beat, digestion, small muscular movements and so on. In a discussion on heat illness, these can be ignored for practical

144

purposes, as the amount of heat produced is small. The principal sources of heat gain which may give rise to heat illness are, therefore,

(*i*) heat from the *environment*, and

(*ii*) heat from *physical work*, due to heat production in muscles. Hard physical work leads to the production of large amounts of heat.

Heat loss

Heat loss from the body takes place by

radiation,
convection,
conduction, and by
evaporation.

In conditions where severe heat stress is present, that is, where the body may have difficulty in getting rid of heat, evaporation of sweat is usually *by far* the most important mechanism for heat loss. For heat to be lost by evaporation, *sweat* must be

—produced, and

— evaporated.

Sweat production

Sweat is normally produced when body temperature rises or tends to rise. The sensing of a rise in body temperature, and the decision to start sweat production, are controlled by the brain. If brain control fails to function, sweat production may cease. A very sharp rise in body temperature—for example, to above 39·5°C (103°F)—may upset brain function, which in turn can lead to inadequate production of sweat and thus to failure of this important heat-losing mechanism. This, or something like it in a more complex way, is thought to be the mechanism of heat illness (*hyperpyrexia*). If no sweat is produced, heat loss by evaporation of sweat ceases, and body temperature may go on rising until death results.

Sweat production may also fail when heat stroke supervenes if inadequate amounts of fluid (water) are present.

Evaporation of sweat

Evaporation of sweat can only take place if the humidity (moisture content) of the surrounding atmosphere permits uptake of more water vapour. Conditions of *high humidity* may therefore make heat loss by sweat evaporation difficult or impossible.

Lack of air movement may also reduce evaporation of sweat. Heavy and *unsuitable clothing* can trap sweat and thus limit evaporation.

THE PREVENTION OF HEAT ILLNESS

Acclimatization plays a very important part in most people, when dealing with the effects of heat. Many cases of heat illness occur in people who are unaccustomed to heat, who are suddenly exposed to heat and who often know little of the precautions which should be taken.

Remembering that radiation, convection, conduction and evaporation are the mechanisms of heat loss, all possible means should be used to aid these processes. As the environmental temperature rises, the possible loss of heat by radiation, convection and conduction decreases, and evaporation by sweating is then the only way of losing heat.

In warm places, heat loss should therefore be encouraged by wearing light clothing to allow heat to be conducted and radiated if possible, and to allow any air movement to cause convection. Evaporation of sweat is also easier on bare or lightly covered areas.

Because sweat consists mainly of salt and water (1·0–3·0 g salt per litre), adequate intakes of both salt and water must be maintained.

People who are exposed to hot environments will probably require *at least* 3·5 litres (6½ pints of fluid per day). Under certain conditions of desert heat, voluntary intakes of fluid up to 14·4 litres (26 pints) per day are not unusual! Extra salt should be taken with food. It may also be wise to take about one saltspoonful of salt with each half pint of fluid, in order to be sure of an adequate salt intake. In case there is any doubt about the size of a saltspoon, we give the Medical Research Council recommendation—one gram of salt per litre of fluid (1 g/litre). Salt *should not* be taken if water supplies are inadequate.

In summary, therefore, exposure to a heat stressing environment should be preceded if possible by acclimatization. Clothing should be light and all available means should be taken to encourage air movement over the skin to allow heat loss by radiation, by convection and by evaporation. Fluid intake should be high—at least 3·5 litres (6½ pints) per day. Salt intake should be stepped up slightly on food, and if hard physical work is done, a saltspoonful of salt should be taken with each half pint of fluid. These amounts should be adequate to prevent salt depletion.

HEAT ILLNESS (SALT/FLUID DEPLETION)

Heat illness (salt/fluid depletion) usually comes on over a period of days. Fatigue is very characteristic of the illness and headache, giddiness and muscle cramps may be felt. If these are ignored, or the reason for them is not apparent, a more acute attack of the illness may follow, characterized by sudden onset with collapse and paleness. Muscle cramps are due to salt depletion and are absent if the cause of the illness is water depletion.

The casualty may vomit. The *skin*, however, will be moist and the casualty's *temperature* will probably not be above 37·8°C (100°F). Heat illness due to salt/fluid depletion is less serious than heat illness (hyperpyrexia), which is described below.

147

HEAT ILLNESS (HYPERPYREXIA)

The exact cause of heat illness (hyperpyrexia) is not known, but it is probably due to a sequence of events as follows.

—Body temperature rises (hot environment, heavy work and so on).

—The heat control centre in the brain fails.

—Sweating fails.

—Various organs of the body suffer heat damage.

This illness usually comes on more rapidly than heat illness (*salt/fluid depletion*) and may or may not be preceded by diminished or absent sweating and by thirst, drowsiness and giddiness. The casualty may vomit. *Mental confusion* followed by *delirium* and *loss of consciousness* occur as body temperature rises. The duration of unconsciousness is important in determining the outcome—longer periods of unconsciousness are associated with higher death rates.

Convulsions and death may follow. Temperatures of 43·3°C (110°F) are usually fatal and *any temperature above 38·9°C (102°F) is an indication that emergency cooling must begin AT ONCE*.

Table 4.1 gives some of the points which distinguish the

TABLE 4.1

	Heat illness (salt/fluid lack)	Heat illness (hyperpyrexia)
Acclimatization	Often unacclimatized	Variable
Salt intake	Low	Normal
Warning of onset	Often present over 2 days	Sometimes present over a shorter time
Cramp	Usual	Unusual
Loss of consciousness	Perhaps	Often
Mental confusion	Not present	Present
Skin	Always moist	Moist or dry
Temperature	37·8°C (100°F) or below	38·3°C (101°F) OR ABOVE

two forms of heat illness. ALWAYS take the TEMPERA-TURE of any casualty whom you think may be suffering from any form of heat illness. If the temperature is above 38·9°C (102°F) start cooling the casualty AT ONCE.

The AIMS of the FIRST-AID TREATMENT of HEAT ILLNESS

Depending on the type of heat illness, the aims will vary, but in general, the aims will be to

—cool the casualty, and

—replace fluid and salt.

Any casualty who is unconscious from heat illness should be treated in the usual way for unconsciousness and, in addition, should be cooled. No fluids should be given by mouth to unconscious casualties. Intravenous fluid and salt replacement can, of course, be given by a doctor or other suitably trained person.

Any casualty thought to be suffering from heat illness should, if possible, be removed at once from the hot environment and placed in a cool or air-conditioned place. If this is not possible, cooling should begin by any available method (*see* later) if the cause is thought to be heat illness (*hyperpyrexia*).

THE FIRST-AID TREATMENT OF HEAT ILLNESS

Heat illness (salt/fluid depletion)

Mild cases of heat illness (salt/fluid depletion), after removal from the hot environment, should be treated by giving *large amounts of fluid*—cool or cold if possible—containing half a level *teaspoonful* of salt in 1 litre (1·8 pints) of water, repeated during the day. Citrus fruit juice flavouring (orange, lemon, lime) is a useful method of disguising the taste of salt in these drinks. Larger amounts of salt can lead to vomiting, thus causing salt and fluid loss and further depletion. Salt should *not* be given alone. Always give salt with plenty of fluid. Mild cooling is also beneficial. The casualty should be kept at rest until he feels better, and for some time after this. An adequate salt/fluid intake should then be ensured to prevent recurrence. In mild cases, response to treatment is usually dramatic and gratifying.

In more severe cases ('heat exhaustion'), after removing the casualty from the heat, give cool salt drinks as described above. In addition, arrange if possible for a doctor to give intravenous saline (salt and fluid) on the spot. If this is not possible, transfer the casualty to hospital.

In any case, check the casualty's temperature to make sure that he is not suffering from heat illness (*hyperpyrexia*). Make written records of the amounts of salt and fluids which the casualty has taken.

When salt/fluid depletion is thought to be the cause of the casualty's heat illness and the casualty *fails to respond* to replacement of salt and fluid, he will be found to be suffering from heat illness (*hyperpyrexia*). This mistake can be avoided by checking the casualty's temperature at an early stage, and by using the other points given in Table 4.1, which differentiate the two forms of heat illness.

Heat illness (hyperpyrexia)

The onset of heat illness (hyperpyrexia) may result in a *serious medical emergency,* requiring prompt treatment of the casualty. If a rise in temperature remains unchecked or rises further, the casualty can easily die or suffer serious effects.

The treatment of heat illness (hyperpyrexia) is to COOL the casualty as RAPIDLY as possible, until the temperature drops to 38·9°C (102°F) or just below. Further cooling should then maintain this temperature. Excessive cooling below this can lead to collapse.

A careful watch must be kept to make sure that the temperature does not rise again. Relapses occur readily.

How cooling is carried out will depend on individual circumstances, but in any case it should be RAPID. The casualty should be stripped naked and placed in the coolest spot within easy access—air-conditioned if possible. Tepid sponging, fanning to increase air movement or any other appropriate measure to reduce body temperature should be taken QUICKLY. The temperature should be taken using a thermometer (*Figure 4.1*) and recorded at 5 minute intervals until 38·9°C (102°F) is reached, and after this, at about 10 minute intervals if the general condition improves. The casualty should then be put to bed and watched carefully. Frequent checks should be made on the general condition of the patient and on his temperature using a thermometer because he may still require further cooling.

Medical help should always be sought.

If the casualty is unconscious he should be treated as any unconscious casualty by placing him in the unconscious position, by making sure that the airway is clear, and by maintaining slight head extension.

If the casualty is conscious, salt-containing cool drinks should be given as detailed earlier.

The casualty should *not* be sent to hospital until his body temperature remains below 38·9°C (102°F) and his general condition has improved. There should also be assurance that there will be no risk of further overheating on the way to hospital—this would undo any good that has been done. Heat illness *(hyperpyrexia)* is an illness in which good first aid can save lives.

Medical first-aid treatment may include alcohol sponging to reduce the body temperature quickly. It is important also to prevent shivering during cooling procedures because shivering generates body heat. Chlorpromazine intramuscularly in a dose of 40–60 mg will prevent shivering.

How to take the temperature

(1) Make sure that the thermometer has been reset by shaking the mercury down until it registers 36°C (97°F) or below.

(2) In adults and older children, the mercury-containing bulb of the thermometer should be placed under the tongue. The lips are then closed. The subject should keep the mouth shut and should not speak while the thermometer is registering the temperature.

In children the thermometer should be placed in the skin fold under the arm or at the top of the leg in the groin. The arm should be held gently into the side or the leg held slightly bent in order to keep the thermometer in contact with the skin *and* to prevent any injury to the child as a result of breaking the thermometer.

(3) After 2 minutes—timed by the clock if possible—the temperature on the thermometer should be read. No error will be caused by leaving the thermometer in for a longer time but with too short a time, the thermometer will indicate too low a temperature.

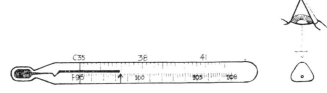

Figure 4.1.—Reading a clinical thermometer

(4) After use, rinse the thermometer in *cold* water to which antiseptic has been added. Never use hot water.

Care is necessary in handling clinical thermometers. If they are dropped or jarred, accuracy will be affected.

THE LOCAL EFFECTS OF HEAT

BURNS AND SCALDS

PREVENTION

The majority of serious burns occur at home to children, elderly frail people and people handicapped by illness or accident. Children are most at risk as they have not learned the dangers of fire and are exploring their environment. In order to protect these three groups and prevent burns, their environment must be made safe and must remain safe.

By far the greatest part—about 90 per cent of the deaths which follow burning injuries at home—are due to clothes catching fire and burning. Although a naked child in contact with flames may suffer deep local burns, the contrast in the number of deaths from burns *without* clothing on fire (3 per cent) and the number of deaths from burns *with* clothing on fire (23 per cent) shows clearly the need to prevent clothes catching fire.

Sources of danger such as naked flames, for example, coal fires, must be securely guarded. Butane camping stoves when alight have flames which are *invisible* in daylight. Many children are burned every summer because they do not see flames and do not realize that the stove is alight. Matches should be kept well out of reach of all children, and children's clothing, especially nightdresses, should be made of non-inflammable materials. Pyjamas, although not as pretty, are much safer than nightdresses. Other common causes of burning at or near home are inflammable liquids, petrol and paraffin, bonfires and fireworks. Burn injuries cause much misery, most of which is clearly preventable. It is our duty to ensure prevention of these injuries.

MEDICAL INFORMATION

Burns from dry heat or wet heat cause skin destruction and damage. The extent of skin destruction is a summation of

—the *thickness* or *depth* of skin burned, and

—the *area* of skin burned.

In first-aid, the most important guide to the severity of a burn is the AREA of skin burned.

SKIN DESTRUCTION BY THICKNESS OR DEPTH

Skin destruction, by thickness or depth, is classified as follows (*Figure 4.2*):

(*i*) superficial skin loss
(*ii*) partial thickness skin loss
(*iii*) total thickness skin loss or whole thickness skin loss.

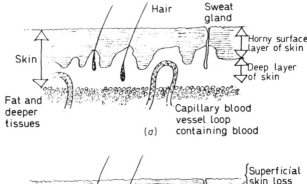

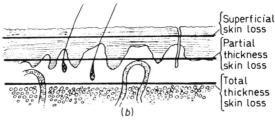

Figure 4.2.—(a) Diagram of skin. (b) Depths of skin loss. (i) A burn causing superficial skin loss (redness only) will extend for a short distance beyond the surface layers of the skin. (ii) A burn causing partial skin loss will extend into the deeper layers of the skin but will spare the ends of the hair follicles and sweat glands. Note that the deep skin–fat border is uneven. Regrowth of skin to cover burned areas will occur from the skin which is spared at the bottom of hair follicles and sweat glands and from the natural dips in the skin–fat junction. (iii) A burn causing total skin loss will extend into the fatty layer (iii) or more deeply (iv).

(*i*) *Superficial skin loss* occurs in mild sunburn and in some flash burns. These burns show redness without blistering and without loss of feeling in the burned areas. Although this type of burn is very painful, the skin is not seriously damaged and will soon get back to normal, provided further damage does not occur.

(*ii*) *Partial thickness skin loss* occurs in many burns. The skin is destroyed down to the deeper layers—but these deep layers remain intact. Skin can then grow out from the islands of skin which survive and cover the denuded areas. This type of skin destruction is often accompanied by blistering and by weeping from burned areas which do not form blisters. There may be a very slight loss of feeling, but a pinprick will usually be clearly felt in the burned area. This type of skin loss requires skilled medical assessment and treatment.

(*iii*) *Total thickness skin loss* is a serious matter. The protective layer of the body is gone and can only be replaced by skin grafting or by ingrowth of skin from the edges of the burned area. Ingrowth of skin is a very slow process—some 1–2 millimetres a week is often the rate of progress. In burns which result in total thickness skin loss, deeper structures may also be burned, such as muscles, bones, blood vessels and so on. The nerve endings which conduct pain sensation are also destroyed. This is why severe burns are often painful at the edges only.

Skin replacement is the best treatment for skin loss.

In burns which cause *superficial skin loss,* skin will be replaced naturally and, due to the slight amount of damage to the skin, there will be little danger of infection.

Where *partial thickness skin loss* occurs, the skin will regenerate itself, provided that it can do so. If infection occurs, skin replacement may be a long and difficult process.

In cases of *total thickness skin loss,* skin replacement by grafting will be required. For skin grafting to be done, there must be enough undamaged skin to provide a donor area and the site where the graft is going to be placed must be in a suitable state to receive a graft. Amongst other things, this means that the area must not be or become infected.

Variable thicknesses of skin may be lost in one incident

Although burns have been described as those which cause superficial skin loss, partial thickness skin loss and total thickness skin loss, different thicknesses of skin loss will often occur following one injury. The edges of a scald, for example, may show redness only corresponding to an area of superficial skin loss. Towards the middle, blistering may occur over an area of partial thickness skin loss, and in the centre of the scalded area where most heat was delivered to the skin, there may be areas of total thickness skin loss.

SKIN DESTRUCTION BY THE AREA WHICH IS BURNED

The remarks which we have made about the thickness of skin destruction will influence the local medical treatment of the burn. It should, however, be re-emphasized here that the seriousness of any burn depends mainly on the AREA of skin which is burned, and not on the thickness or depth of skin destruction.

Burns which are large in area will tend to give rise to greater body fluid loss than burns which affect a small area, even if the latter are relatively deeper. The general effect of burns, which in the early stages is mainly due to plasma and fluid loss, will therefore tend to be worse in proportion to the percentage of body surface which is damaged.

It is possible to arrive at a quick assessment of the percentage of body surface which is burned by the use of the 'rule of nines'. *Figure 4.3* shows the way in which the body is divided into skin areas with multiples of 9. A skin area the size of *the casualty's* hand is roughly 1 per cent of the body surface.

In adults, burns of 15 per cent or more may need plasma transfusion, burns of over 20 per cent will probably require

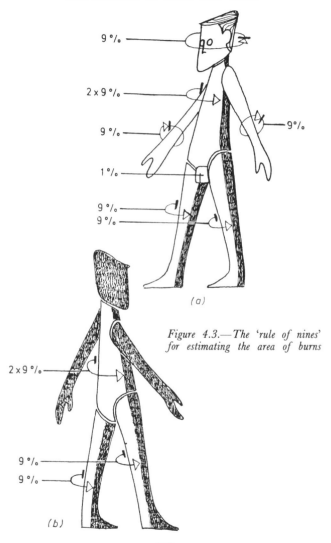

Figure 4.3.—The 'rule of nines' for estimating the area of burns

plasma and over 25 per cent will certainly require plasma. Burns of 45 per cent or more will give rise to serious medical treatment problems, and burns of over 75 per cent will usually be fatal. In children and in old people, burns of much smaller areas will be more serious and will require transfusion.

FLUID LOSS IN BURNS

When skin or other tissue is damaged, body fluids can leak out through the damaged areas. This gives rise to blisters or to weeping *(Figure 4.4)*. The composition of this

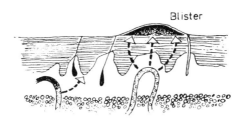

Figure 4.4.—Fluid escapes through damaged skin and blood vessels

fluid is roughly equivalent to the liquid part of blood, the plasma. As a result of this fluid loss, there are more blood cells in a given volume of blood, and the blood is therefore thicker and the cells more concentrated. A considerable protein loss occurs in this fluid loss.

Fluid replacement is therefore an aim of first-aid burn treatment. The best replacement for the plasma which is lost is plasma given intravenously. This cannot often be given except in hospitals. In first-aid for fluid loss in burns give small quantities of water, or of other bland fluid, until the casualty reaches hospital. In a conscious adult, not more than half a cup of water every 10 minutes should be given. Greater quantities may lead to vomiting. No fluid should be given by mouth to unconscious casualties.

Children who are conscious should be given much smaller amounts of water, fizzy drinks or other bland fluid, by mouth.

Remember that *no* fluids should be given by mouth to unconscious casualties.

Burn casualties are likely to remain conscious if they are suffering only from burns. Unconsciousness, except in very severe burns—50 per cent or more of the body surface burned—will probably be due to other injuries.

The AIMS of FIRST-AID for BURNS
(1) Prevent further damage by immediate cooling.
(2) Prevent infection.
(3) Minimize the effects of fluid loss from the burned tissues.
(4) Reassure the burned person.
(5) Transport the casualty swiftly to hospital. *See New Essential First-Aid* for further details of first-aid for burns.

COOLING FOR BURNS

The acceptance of cooling as a useful treatment for burns is still far from universal, and we are therefore including a few words about why cooling can and should be used, together with some references to published work on the subject.

Just as an egg will go on cooking after it has been removed from boiling water, so can a heat burn 'go on cooking' and continue to increase in severity until the temperature falls. The quickest way to accomplish a fall in temperature is to cool the burned area as quickly as possible following injury. Cooling should be continued for 10 minutes timed by the clock—long enough to accomplish this desired fall in temperature, but not for so long that the casualty's arrival in hospital will be seriously delayed. Clothing, which is not stuck, should be removed during cooling as clothing can retain heat. This is particularly important following scalding. Do not attempt to remove clothing which is stuck to skin following heat burns. Much good skin can be stripped off in this way to the detriment of the casualty.

Burns and scalds first cause pain and tissue damage, then loss of blood plasma into the tissues surrounding damaged capillaries, and may stop effective blood supply to the burned area.

Much work has demonstrated beyond reasonable doubt that immediate cooling not only arrests further thermal injury but minimizes the resultant loss of tissue and skin damage from a heat burn or scald. If clean cool water is to hand, showering or immersion relieves pain drastically and takes less time than producing sterile dressings of the right size. Ten minutes spent cooling a burn will not significantly affect the hospital treatment of a burn, but it may greatly affect the amount and depth of local thermal injury. Local cooling is an effective and readily available first-aid procedure, and may be the only means of providing first-aid treatment in mass casualties.

THE GENERAL EFFECTS OF COLD

ACUTE HYPOTHERMIA

Immersion chilling
Wet–cold chilling (exposure)

IMMERSION CHILLING

Many deaths from 'drowning' are not due to water in the lungs and inability to breathe, but are caused by the lowering of body temperature due to immersion in cold water, that is, by *immersion chilling* (immersion hypothermia). It is estimated that there are about 1,000 lives lost every year around the coasts of Great Britain from immersion chilling amongst dinghy sailors and the victims of shipwreck. When the liner 'Laconia' sank north of Madeira about 113 out of 124 deaths were thought to be due to immersion chilling. The mean sea-water temperature on the day before and after the disaster was 17·9°C (64·2°F); the mean air temperature on the same days was 15·7°C (60·3°F); and the sea temperature was not lower at night than 17°C (62·6°F). *See* the diagram on page 164 for survival times.

A naked man will lose about 27 times as much heat in water at 1·1–1·6°C (34–35°F) than in still air at the same temperature.

MEDICAL INFORMATION

Studies of immersion chilling have shown that below 10°C (50°F), blood vessels lose their ability to shut off blood flow by contracting, and therefore heat is lost through the skin.

At 10°C and above, most people can maintain body temperature. At slightly higher water temperatures, people with less fat can maintain their body temperature. The only individual factor which affects ability to maintain body temperature during cold water immersion is body fat thickness. Fat acts as a layer of insulation. Studies have also shown that when a person is immersed in cold water and body temperature cannot be maintained, work and exercise is *always harmful*. Activity of any kind, such as swimming, causes movement of cold water over and around

TABLE 4.2

The average fall in rectal temperature in °C after immersion for 20 minutes in water at 5°C

		°C
No work	Unclothed	1·23
Moderate work	Unclothed	1·81
Hard work	Unclothed	1·61
Working	Clothed	0·61
No work	Clothed	0·29

the body surface and therefore results in greater heat loss. It has also been shown that clothing delays the fall in body temperature. Clothing acts as an insulator.

The figures in Table 4.2, from work by Dr W. R. Keatinge, show the fall in basal body temperature (rectal temperature) which is experienced, under differing conditions of clothing and work, during immersion for 20 minutes in water at 5°C (41°F). In the course of the experiment, 600 immersions were made in cold water by naval volunteers. These figures show that the least fall in basic body temperature occurs in those who are clothed and who remain at rest.

THE PREVENTION OF IMMERSION CHILLING

Do not get into cold water

Attention to water safety rules could prevent many needless immersions in cold water. It may appear to be stating the obvious to say 'do not get into cold water' but many people still approach water sports without an adequate knowledge of water safety, seamanship or the study of local weather conditions. Neglect of elementary safety rules and lack of foresight are still common causes of immersion. Other occasions such as capsize or shipwreck may occur, which are beyond the control of the individual.

It is important to distinguish between the quick immersion which may be required to rescue a person from drowning— which should not normally lead to immersion chilling— and the other occasions when people get into cold water and may have to stay there until rescued or for some unforeseeable amount of time. It is for the latter cases, where immersion chilling may be a problem, that we offer the advice below.

Wear as much clothing as possible before getting into the water

If the clothing is wind and waterproof, so much the better. This will delay wetting and will trap a still layer of air or water next to the skin when soaking does occur. In this way body heat will be less well conducted into the surrounding cold water and chilling will therefore be delayed. A 'wet suit' is an application of this principle.

Keep still in the water

Heat loss is minimized by stillness: swimming, treading water or doing exercise to generate body heat merely result in greater heat loss.

Many intelligent people, used to thinking of conditions which favour keeping warm *in air*, might think that exercise and swimming would generate heat and thus delay whole body chilling during immersion. This is not so in water. Swimming and movement do generate heat, but the heat gain is small by comparison with the greatly increased heat loss arising from water movement round the body. *The net result is that movement increases chilling*. This fact requires to be much more widely appreciated and acted upon.

The immersion casualty

People who are immersed in cold water may suffer from two conditions

—*drowning* (not breathing due to water)

—*hypothermia* (wet-cold chilling)

The likely survival time of any person in cold water will depend on two main considerations

—the temperature of the water

—the clothing worn

The amount of body fat, which acts as insulation, will also affect survival time. The elderly and the very young do not tolerate cold.

Low water temperatures and flimsy or absent clothing will allow only short survival times. Thin people will become chilled more quickly than fat people.

This means that 50 per cent of people in the water around the U.K., even in the summer, become unconscious within two hours.

163

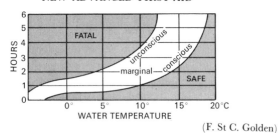

(F. St C. Golden)

Approximate life expectancy in water in normal clothes

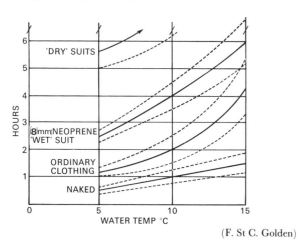

(F. St C. Golden)

Estimated time of useful consciousness of differently clothed people in cold water (estimated under laboratory conditions)

The AIMS of FIRST-AID for IMMERSION CASUALTIES are to

— *rescue* the casualty as soon as possible.
— *give artificial respiration* if not breathing.
— *give heart compression* if the heart has stopped.
— *insulate* the casualty to prevent further heat loss.

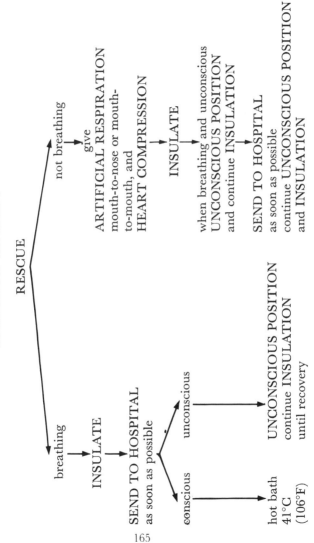

Summary of first-aid for the
IMMERSION CASUALTY

RESCUE

breathing → INSULATE → SEND TO HOSPITAL
as soon as possible

conscious → hot bath 41°C (106°F)

unconscious → UNCONSCIOUS POSITION continue INSULATION until recovery

not breathing → give ARTIFICIAL RESPIRATION mouth-to-nose or mouth-to-mouth, and HEART COMPRESSION

INSULATE

when breathing and unconscious UNCONSCIOUS POSITION and continue INSULATION

SEND TO HOSPITAL as soon as possible continue UNCONSCIOUS POSITION and INSULATION

165

Details of first-aid for not breathing are given on page 16, for heart compression page 6, and for unconsciousness page 4. Wet-cold chilling is discussed on page 166.

Insulation of the casualty should be accomplished as quickly as possible by removing the casualty to a sheltered place if possible and then wrapping him in warm blankets. Care should be taken in removing clothing lest further chilling takes place. If in doubt, insulate on top of wet clothing. In the open, place the casualty in a large polythene sack and insulate this (see wet-cold chilling, page 166).

Conscious casualties should be put in a hot bath at 41°C (106°F), leaving the legs and arms out of the water whenever possible. This will prevent the cold blood in the arms and legs entering the body and lowering the body or core temperature. The bathroom should be very warm to ensure the casualty breathes warm moist air to prevent heat loss from the respiratory tract.

A note about deaths from 'drowning'

Many deaths which are said to be due to drowning have nothing to do with inability to breathe or with water in the lungs; they are due to hypothermia in the form of immersion chilling. The prevention of deaths from drowning is usually thought of in terms of keeping afloat, and most survival equipment caters only for this important need. There is, however, an additional need in many instances— that of keeping warm in cold water. The importance of trying to prevent immersion chilling should not be forgotten by those who devise safety rules for 'drowning prevention'.

WET-COLD CHILLING

An acute form of chilling, wet–cold chilling, which arises in presumably fit adults or young people is an important cause of deaths on the mountains and in open country. Adequate equipment, including waterproof clothing and overgarments, skilled leadership, reasonable fitness and common-sense use of local knowledge and weather forecasts would prevent most cases of wet–cold chilling. If any person shows a likelihood of becoming wet or tired, shelter should be sought *at once*. When a person shows any early signs of wet–cold chilling such as abnormal behaviour, slow responses, excessive tiredness or apathy and weakness or stumbling, the surest way to prevent disaster is to camp. Wet–cold chilling casualties should be treated by being *dried* and *heated*. (*See New Essential First Aid*, Pan, 1984.)

A few additional words about prevention

In the prevention of wet–cold chilling, the effects of head and face covering should never be forgotten. About 20 per cent of the heat from the body can be lost in this way, whilst the rest of the body is clothed. Fur and leather helmets, sou'westers and balaclavas have all an important role in prevention of heat loss from these areas. A large hooded cape (cagoule) is also a valuable piece of equipment, as this can be used to 'camp' in by crouching in a position of shelter whilst wearing the cape.

An extra note about rewarming in wet–cold chilling

Always try to revive the apparently dead following exposure on the mountains and in similar conditions of chilling by wet–cold. Make sure that blankets do not cover the faces and mouths of such casualties to ensure that they can breathe. They may be alive, even though breathing is not easy to detect under adverse conditions. The task of a first-aider is to act in order to save lives: he should *not* assume that a casualty is dead as a result of an inadequate examination under adverse conditions, for example, on a snowy mountain-side. All such casualties should be treated as alive until a doctor pronounces them to be dead. Widely dilated pupils should also be disregarded as a sign of death. Such casualties may be very near to the point of death, but they may also be capable of being revived by rewarming.

Carry them in a head-low position to a place where re-warming can be performed. Until rewarming has been carried out, it is always best to hope that the casualty can be revived and to aim to carry out rewarming at the earliest opportunity. Always attempt treatment until a doctor rules that it is of no further use. Lives can be saved in this way.

SUBACUTE OR CHRONIC HYPOTHERMIA— CHILLING IN BABIES AND OLD PEOPLE

MEDICAL INFORMATION

A less acute form of chilling can occur in people who are *more susceptible* to the effects of cold, that is, in babies and in old people. In both of these groups, the heat regulating mechanism of the body functions less well than in adults and young people and as a result they may be overcome *gradually* by cold.

A typical instance is that of the baby or old person who is found unconscious in a cold room. In the case of young babies, the blankets and bedding may have been kicked off. The appearance of the casualty in each case is similar—unconscious, pale, perhaps even moribund, and COLD to the touch in an environment which is cold or below about 18°C (64°F).

PREVENTION

Babies—especially in the first 4 months of life—and old people should, if possible, remain in a warm environment. Bedrooms are often cold and it is here that chilling occurs. *The prevention of chilling is mainly a matter of staying in a warm environment rather than heaping on clothes and blankets in a cold room.* It is the cold environment which leads to chilling. Any room in which a young baby is left should be kept at around 21°C (70°F). Old people living alone—often in poverty—are the usual victims of chilling. Inadequate environmental warmth, combined at times with insufficiently nourishing food and lowered body-heat production, allows these old people to succumb to chilling in temperatures which would not affect normal healthy adults.

Prevention is largely a matter of adequate environmental warmth—19–21°C (66–70°F)—adequate diet, and some supervision of old people living alone to make sure that they are seen to be going about their normal routines. Some cases of chilling have not been discovered until the old person has been in a chilled state for 2 days. This sort of tragedy can be averted or greatly lessened by neighbourliness.

Close the bedroom window and keep it closed if it is cold.

The AIMS of FIRST-AID for CHILLING in BABIES and OLD PEOPLE

(1) Prevent further heat loss, but do not rewarm.
(2) Send the baby or old person swiftly to hospital.
It should be noted that first-aid for the slower onset type of chilling which occurs in babies and old people is *different* from the treatment of the sudden chilling which occurs in fit adults.

PREVENT FURTHER HEAT LOSS BUT DO NOT REWARM

Cover the casualty with the *normal amount* of blankets which would be used by a fit adult in the temperature of the surroundings in which you find the casualty. That is, prevent further heat loss, but do no more than this.

MAKE NO EFFORTS TO REWARM THE BABY OR OLD PERSON

—Do NOT cover with a heap of blankets.
—Do NOT use electric blankets or hot water bottles.
—Do NOT heat the room by any means.
—Do NOT give hot drinks.

—Do NOT attempt to rewarm the baby or old person by immersing him in a hot bath or by immersing the limbs in a sink or bucket.

Make sure the baby or old person is resting on warm blankets.

SEND THE BABY OR OLD PERSON SWIFTLY TO HOSPITAL

Babies can be taken to hospital by car. Old people will usually require an ambulance.

The reasons for the differences in treatment of immersion and wet–cold chilling on the one hand and chilling in babies and old people on the other are fairly complex, but are concerned with differences in the rates of onset, the results of rapid or slow temperature drops, and the ease or difficulty in reversal of these changes.

THE LOCAL EFFECT OF COLD

FROSTBITE

MEDICAL INFORMATION

Frostbite is a type of tissue damage due to cold which occurs mainly in the extremities, for example, the hands and feet, or in exposed parts such as the ears and nose. Frostbite can, however, occur elsewhere. In extreme cases, due to localized heat loss and chilling, actual freezing of tissues may occur. At first, the frozen area is pale, due to the stopping of the circulation of blood through the area. Initially there may be only a feeling of cold followed by pain. The part later becomes blue and, when thawing occurs, blisters may form. In developed frostbite, the part is numb, stiff and lifeless, but intense pain is unusual.

TABLE 4.3

Immersion and wet–cold chilling (acute hypothermia)	Chilling in babies and old people (subacute or chronic hypothermia)
Occurs in fit adults or young people who are *NOT specially susceptible* to cold	Occurs in babies and old people who are *specially susceptible* to cold
The onset of *chilling* is usually *rapid* or *very rapid*	The onset of *chilling* is usually *moderate, slow* or *very slow*
The changes due to rapid chilling *can be reversed by rapid rewarming*	The changes due to slow chilling can be made much worse by rapid rewarming. Therefore *slow or very slow rewarming is required* in hospital, together with other special treatment

PREVENTION

Prevention is the obvious course to follow. Those who are exposed to a cold environment are usually aware of the hazard of frostbite and should wear adequate loose-fitting clothing, and should practise meticulous standards of personal hygiene. Before going into a cold environment the skin should be thoroughly dry, as moisture increases heat loss and thus increases the chance of frostbite.

Early symptoms of frostbite, when the casualty is suffering from *superficial frostbite*, are a feeling of cold or numbness, most often in hands and fingers, feet and toes, or nose and ears. These early symptoms should always be heeded so that treatment can start immediately. Later signs and symptoms of *deep frostbite* are coldness, complete lack of feeling in the part, whiteness or blueness of the part—indicating lack of circulation—and stiffness.

Frostbite, like wet–cold chilling, occurs most frequently when people are tired, careless or in some way incapacitated by injuries, sickness, excessive fatigue or unconsciousness.

171

In severe wintry conditions, loss of a glove can easily lead to frostbite. It is therefore wise to carry spares of certain items such as gloves and socks. If a glove is lost and a spare glove is not available, socks or scarves should be used to protect the hand. Lack of covering will lead to much faster heat loss from the part and therefore to local chilling and frostbite.

The AIMS of FIRST-AID for FROSTBITE

(1) Rewarm the frostbitten part.
(2) Prevent infection and further injury after rewarming.
(3) Get the casualty to hospital.

Many casualties who are frostbitten (a local effect of cold) are also chilled (hypothermic) (a general effect of cold) and may also have other injuries. *All* of these conditions will require appropriate assessment and treatment.

All casualties suffering from frostbite should go, or be taken, to the nearest place where adequate rewarming can be carried out as quickly as possible (*see* later).

Rings or tight clothing such as boots which tend to constrict the part should be loosened or removed (*Figures 4.5 and 4.6*).

TREATMENT

Frostbite can be divided into two categories:
— superficial frostbite (frost nip) and
— deep frostbite.

Superficial frostbite

Very mild frostbite, or superficial frostbite—sometimes called 'frost nip'—is the only type which can be treated away from special facilities. The affected part should be treated by removing clothing and by rewarming it against another warm part of the body—for example, an affected hand can be placed in the opposite arm-pit. It

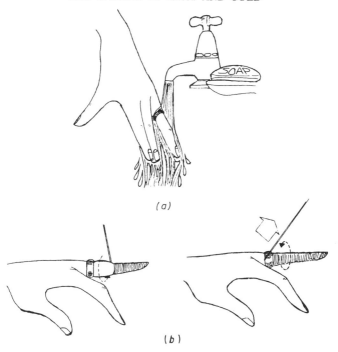

(a)

(b)

Figure 4.5.—(a) A ring may slip easily off a wet soapy finger. (b) Another method of removing a tight ring

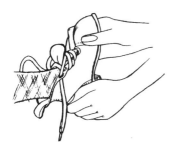

Figure 4.6.—Gently remove tight clothing and boots

may be necessary to rewarm feet by using another person's body heat. The casualty places his foot on a warm part of the other person, say in the arm-pit or on the back. The nose or ears can be covered by cupped hands.

Deep frostbite

With deep frostbite the part(s) should be rewarmed in water at 40–44°C (104–111°F). Higher temperatures can do harm by burning.

Treatment should *not* begin until adequate facilities are at hand. Contrary to popular belief, a person can probably walk on frostbitten feet for some distance without seriously injuring his feet, and may be wise to do so in order to reach a place where proper treatment can be carried out. *Once rewarming has begun, no further weight bearing or walking should be allowed as this will then increase the damage.* Similarly, after rewarming, exercise in order to stimulate the circulation should be forbidden as this will only increase the area of damage and loss. Rubbing with snow or anything else is useless and harmful; it should be forbidden. Smoking should not be allowed as tobacco causes the blood vessels in some people to narrow and stop the circulation of blood through them.

Alcohol in limited quantities may be useful during the rewarming period only, because alcohol causes small blood vessels to dilate, and thus increases the flow of blood through them.

Rewarming.—A *large* container should be used for rewarming so that
  (*i*) the water can be kept at the optimal temperature of 40–44°C (104–111°F) and
  (*ii*) the part can be completely immersed.
About 20 minutes at this optimal temperature will usually produce complete rewarming. Higher water temperatures should not be used to speed rewarming because this may do

further harm. Rapid rewarming by this method is a painful procedure and the casualty may require pain-relieving drugs.

After rewarming, dry the part by gentle *patting* with a sterile or clean towel or sheet. Be sure that you do not rub or bruise the frostbitten part.

If water is not available, place the frostbitten part against the warm skin of another person. This procedure will take much longer—possibly about 2 hours—to achieve complete rewarming.

If the above methods of rewarming cannot be used, wrap the part(s) in a blanket.

Beware. In cases of frostbite:

—DO NOT rub the part briskly with the hands or with a towel.

—DO NOT rub snow or anything else on the part.

—DO NOT heat the part in very hot water or in an oven.

—DO NOT allow weight-bearing or walking after rewarming.

—DO NOT attempt to rewarm deep frostbite until adequate facilities are to hand.

People who suffer from frostbite may also be the victims of general chilling (hypothermia), and perhaps other injuries. Casualties who suffer from frostbite should be examined to detect other injuries so that appropriate treatment may be instituted. General chilling—in this case, usually acute hypothermia—should be treated appropriately by rapid rewarming in a hot bath and by hot drinks if the casualty is conscious.

After rewarming.—The rewarmed part should be treated to prevent infection and to prevent any further injury caused perhaps by bumping, crushing or weight-bearing. The part should be loosely wrapped in a sterile sheet—or in the cleanest thing available, such as a freshly laundered pillowcase or towel—and should be placed on a soft pillow or cushion. Prevent bedclothes and blankets from pressing on the rewarmed frostbitten area by using a protective 'cage' over it (*Figure 4.7*). If blisters form, they should be left intact and should not be broken. Broken blisters permit entry of germs and thus lead to infection. Ideally the temperature of the room should be kept between 21–26°C (70–78°F).

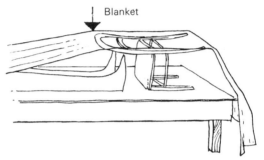

Figure 4.7.—A simple method for keeping blankets off injured feet or legs

When removing the casualty to hospital, particular care should be taken to prevent further damage to the injured part by pressure and weight-bearing. Therefore, ensure that the injured part continues to be kept free of the weight of bedclothes and of tight bandages and dressings.

CHAPTER 5

ILLNESS AND OTHER MEDICAL CONDITIONS

A man who fears suffering is already
suffering for what he fears.
MICHAEL DE MONTAIGNE

ILLNESS

HEART ATTACK

MEDICAL INFORMATION

A heart attack (coronary thrombosis) is due to the heart muscle being suddenly deprived of its blood supply. There is a clot (thrombus) blocking the coronary arteries which supply the heart muscle with blood. Under these conditions, the heart muscle cannot work properly. Depending, therefore, on the amount of muscle which is affected, the casualty may have a heart which is slightly inefficient, moderately inefficient, or so much affected that death results.

A heart attack (coronary thrombosis) may be recognized by the onset of a sudden and usually *severe* pain felt under the left side of the breastbone, which often radiates down the left arm and perhaps to the root of the neck, and may be accompanied by collapse. The casualty is usually a man aged 40–60 years. Occasionally the pain may be described as 'like indigestion'. Heart attacks are about two and a half times more common in cigarette smokers than in non-smokers or cigar smokers.

Casualties who suffer from the pain of a heart attack are sometimes in great fear of death. This fear of death in a casualty who has a sudden onset of severe chest pain usually means that the casualty has had a coronary thrombosis.

Mild heart attacks may make little general change in the casualty's state, but severe attacks will be accompanied by pallor, sweating and general collapse. The pulse is usually weak and may on occasions be irregular.

TREATMENT

Casualties who have suffered a severe heart attack should NOT BE MOVED until they have been seen and treated by a doctor. Until the doctor arrives, *it is essential that the casualty be kept at rest where he is*. He should *not,* for example, be moved upstairs to bed if he is downstairs, or dragged or lifted away from where he is, unless he is in a position of danger. Make him comfortable where he is.

Any physical exertion, *however slight*, will throw extra strain on the heart. Added strain under such conditions may tip the balance in an unfavourable direction. No attempts should therefore be made to rush such a casualty to hospital. Excitement and the effort of moving may make things worse. He should be kept *at rest* where he is until seen and treated by a doctor. *Give oxygen, if available, until the arrival of the doctor* (page 26).

Sudden collapse may, in some cases of heart attacks, be accompanied by stoppage of the heart and stoppage of breathing. Some of these casualties can be successfully resuscitated provided that heart compression and artificial respiration are immediately applied (pages 6 and 16).

Most casualties with a moderate or serious heart attack will be most comfortable in a half-sitting position—the positions used for any casualty who has difficulty in breathing (*Figure 5.1*).

The ambulance ride may be a contributory cause of death in casualties who, following a coronary thrombosis, are rushed into an ambulance and are driven roughly to hospital. There is also some evidence that such casualties should travel half sitting up and *facing the direction of travel,* that is, looking forwards. When facing backwards, the forces acting on the casualty tend to push the diaphragm upwards, thus further embarrassing the action of the heart.

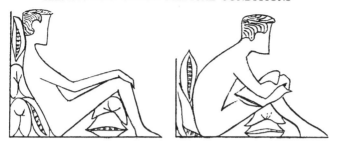

Figure 5.1.—Sitting positions for conscious casualties with difficulty in breathing

Oxygen should be administered continuously in the ambulance to any casualty whose general condition is thought to be affected by the heart attack.

ASTHMA

MEDICAL INFORMATION

Asthma is a condition characterized by episodic difficult, *wheezy* breathing. The onset is usually sudden or fairly rapid in any person who will be a first-aid problem. The casualty will usually appear to be very short of breath and wheezy noises will be heard on approaching him. He will usually be upright or half sitting up to ease breathing. Sufferers from asthma do not lie down when they have a bad attack. On closer observation it will be seen that the casualty has less difficulty in breathing *in* than in breathing *out*.

Sometimes, the casualty will know why an attack has started; on the other hand, he may have no ideas as to why.

Distress may be—and often is—a prominent feature of a severe asthmatic attack. In addition to the difficulty in breathing, the person may feel that he is going to die, or that he has such difficulty in getting his breath that he may not get the next.

179

TREATMENT

Place the casualty at once at rest in the half-sitting positions which ease breathing difficulties (*Figure 5.1*). Reassure him that he is unlikely to come to harm in an attack, and try to calm his panic and his fears that he cannot draw breath easily. Part of the difficulty may be due to panting and panic —and when the casualty can be persuaded to settle down, his breathing may ease. If the casualty is in a cold atmosphere and you can get him into a warm place easily, do this. It may help. If difficulty in breathing is very great, oxygen may be given until the doctor arrives or until the casualty reaches hospital. The most useful first-aid measures, however, are liable to be those concerned with allaying fear and using posture to best advantage.

DIABETES MELLITUS

MEDICAL INFORMATION

Diabetes mellitus—usually abbreviated to diabetes— is due to a disturbance of the mechanisms which control the amount of glucose (sugar) in the blood. The blood glucose is normally kept within certain well defined limits.

THE CONTROL OF THE BLOOD GLUCOSE LEVEL

—The blood glucose level goes *up* following intake of starchy foods, or after eating sugar or things which contain sugar. All of these substances are digested to produce glucose.

—The blood glucose level goes *down* in response to insulin. Insulin is a hormone produced by the pancreas (sweetbread). If the pancreas stops making insulin, the blood glucose level will therefore tend to rise and the person is said to suffer from diabetes.

Normally, the amount of insulin which is produced is sufficient to balance the rise in blood glucose level produced by intake of starchy or sugar-containing food. If insulin is not produced—or is made in too small amounts—the blood glucose level can be controlled by restricting the intake of starchy or sugar-containing foods and/or by injecting insulin. This is how doctors treat people who suffer from diabetes. In place of insulin, certain other drugs can be given to lower the blood glucose level. These are given as tablets, by mouth.

If blood glucose levels stray outside the normally defined limits, two forms of illness can arise.

—The blood glucose level is too *high* (hyperglycaemia*).

—The blood glucose level is too *low* (hypoglycaemia*).

The blood glucose level is too high (hyperglycaemia)

Two forms of onset of high blood glucose levels can be described according to whether the rate of onset is slow or rapid.

Slow onset.—In people who begin to suffer from diabetes, the blood glucose level usually rises at a slow rate. The sufferer may notice increasing thirst and seems to drink excessively. He therefore passes urine more frequently. He then may notice progressive loss of weight followed perhaps by headaches and loss of appetite. His breath may smell of musty apples. If he remains untreated he can become drowsy, unconscious and may die. Unconsciousness due to a raised blood glucose level is usually referred to as *diabetic coma*. The sudden onset of diabetic coma in these circumstances is uncommon if not rare.

Rapid onset.—Although uncommon, diabetic coma can occur suddenly. The casualty is usually a person who is known to suffer from diabetes and who has stopped or forgotten to take his customary dosage of insulin or tablets. The blood glucose level will therefore rise.

---

* hyper—too much; glyc—glucose; aemia—in the blood; hypo—too little.

The blood glucose level is too low (hypoglycaemia)

Lowering of the normal blood glucose level precipitates a medical emergency which is usually *attributed to* and described as insulin overdose. This, however, is misleading and often untrue. Rarely does a diabetic person take more than his normal dose of insulin or tablets. The low blood glucose level is due to *relative overdose* of insulin or tablets, three examples of which follow.

(*i*) The person takes his normal dose of insulin or tablets, but due to incipient infection such as a cold, influenza or simple gastric upset, he does not take any or sufficient food. The balance is therefore destroyed between the intake of food and the amount of insulin or tablets taken.

(*ii*) From an unexpected or prolonged exercise he uses up the available blood glucose as fuel for his muscles.

(*iii*) Due to an unexpected delay in a meal time—perhaps caused by being caught in a traffic jam or even by poor service in a restaurant—his blood glucose level falls below the critical level which is necessary to maintain normal brain function.

The onset of the effect of a low blood glucose level is FAST because glucose is vital for the normal activity of the brain and spinal cord. Characteristically the casualty appears to be drunk and talks meaningless gibberish. Then, if he still remains untreated, he becomes unconscious.

AIDS TO THE EARLY DIAGNOSIS OF A LOW BLOOD GLUCOSE LEVEL

The casualty will

—be a known diabetic; always ask. He may also wear a tag or bracelet.

—have a pale face and skin.

—have a rapid pulse, becoming weaker.

—be sweating, possibly profusely.

—be restless.

—probably show abnormal behaviour; he may resent your offer of help, may stagger or leap about, wave his arms purposelessly, and talk gibberish.

TREATMENT

It is not possible in first-aid to treat a blood glucose level which is too high except by treating unconsciousness in the usual way and by sending the casualty to hospital.

It is an easy matter, however, to treat a blood glucose level which is too low by giving sugar by mouth, *provided that the casualty is conscious* and can therefore be given things by mouth. Sugar by mouth must be given *quickly*, or the casualty may easily become unconscious. If the casualty becomes unconscious, nothing must be given by mouth.

The first-aid treatment of a casualty thought to have a low blood glucose level

Act quickly.

Ensure that the casualty is conscious and can swallow, because nothing must be given by mouth to an unconscious casualty.

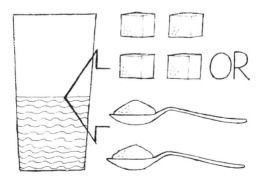

Figure 5.2.—If conscious, give sugar at once

Quickly dissolve 2 to 4 teaspoonsful (or 4 to 8 lumps) of
sugar in about half a glass of water; and persuade the
casualty to drink it (*Figure 5.2*). Granulated sugar or
caster is preferable to lumps, because lumps dissolve
more slowly. Dissolving the sugar in water facilitates
easier and faster absorption and thus helps to prevent
unconsciousness.

If recovery is not swift and complete, give a further amount
of sugar as above.

Persuade the casualty to see a doctor. This step may be
difficult due to the disturbed brain function which
accompanies the condition. Any casualty who has been
suffering from a low blood glucose level *may* need
medical treatment and *will* require medical supervision.

If you are too late and the casualty becomes, or is, unconscious, he should be treated in the usual way for unconsciousness (page 4).

It is possible also to mis-diagnose the casualty's condition.
The reason for his appearance and behaviour may be that
the blood glucose level is too high. In this unlikely event,
it is reassuring to know that, while the extra sugar will not
benefit him, equally *it will do no harm*.

It may also be that the casualty's condition is nothing
whatever to do with diabetes or with his blood glucose level.
However, this should not deter the giving of a sugar-
containing drink to any casualty thought to be suffering
from a low blood glucose level. If the casualty is conscious
and can safely be given a sugar-containing drink, this may
do a great deal of good—and the casualty will be prevented
from becoming unconscious. Where the diagnosis is wrong,
no harm will be done. *The lesson is therefore that if you suspect
a low blood glucose level, always give adequate amounts of sugar
quickly*. No harm will be done in a conscious casualty if
your diagnosis is not correct, but if it is right much good will
have been done.

Speed in giving adequate amounts of sugar is vital if

unconsciousness is to be prevented. After giving sugar, observe the casualty closely for some time. If he again shows signs of deterioration such as sweating, drowsiness or mental confusion, give further amounts of sugar.

Then arrange for the casualty to see a doctor.

Any casualty who has just had an episode of low blood glucose level which requires correction by giving sugar must not be allowed to drive.

PREVENTION

All known sufferers from diabetes should carry a quantity of sugar or glucose sweets with them. Then, if some unforeseen event occurs—simple in itself but which for the person may be life-threatening—he can arrest the fall of his blood glucose level by quickly eating the sugar. A card which clearly states his name, address and the fact that he suffers from diabetes should also be carried—perhaps with instructions such as 'If I am acting strangely, please give me some sugar—2 to 4 heaped teaspoonsful dissolved in water'.

STROKE

MEDICAL INFORMATION

A stroke is an illness which comes on suddenly and is caused by cutting off the blood supply to a part of the brain, or by bleeding into a part of the brain. The sufferer is usually middle-aged or elderly, but may occasionally be a younger person. The extent of the loss of blood supply to the brain or of the bleeding will determine the amount of brain damage, and thus the severity of the stroke. Strokes are not painful in themselves, but may be preceded by severe headaches or a general feeling of being unwell. Brain damage shows mainly by paralysis, that is, by the inability to move some or all of the face, lips, tongue, arms and legs. The paralysis may affect, for example, the whole of one lower limb or may result in some weakness of part of a leg only. If the stroke is a severe one, it will paralyse the arm and leg on one side of the body and the face on the same or on the other side. The casualty may also be unconscious, and, in addition, incontinent, that is, he loses control of his bowel and bladder.

TREATMENT

If the casualty is unconscious, treat him in the usual way for all unconscious casualties and send him to hospital or send for a doctor. Casualties who have had a stroke and seem only partially conscious can often hear and understand what is said to them but cannot reply because the muscles of their tongue and lips are paralysed. So, try to speak to them in such a way that they can make simple signs back to you that they understand what you have said. Casualties who have had a mild stroke, that is, one which results in a small amount of paralysis and following which the casualty is not unconscious, should be put to bed or at rest until a doctor can see them.

Try to reassure any casualty whom you think has had a stroke. Even though the casualty may appear fuddled, he may understand what you say although he is unable to reply. Be careful of what you say in the hearing of such casualties; they often pick up messages which people think they neither hear nor understand.

Although it is said elsewhere (but not in this book) that casualties who have had a stroke should be laid on their backs with their head and shoulders raised, we believe that this is bad advice. ALL unconscious or semi-conscious casualties—including those who have had a stroke—should be placed in the unconscious position, should have the airway cleared of dentures, vomit and so on, and should have a slight head-down tip applied. The prevention of airway obstruction is *by far* the most important aim of first-aid treatment in any casualty whose heart is beating, who is breathing and who is not fully conscious.

EPILEPSY

MEDICAL INFORMATION

About 1 in 200 of the population are epileptic at some time in their lives—so the condition is a common one. It is also one which frequently gives rise to excessive fear in both sufferers and relatives.

The characteristic feature of the condition is that the person suffers from a fit or convulsion. In a typical fit, the casualty loses consciousness, and he may appear to hold his breath and go slightly stiff. As a result of this momentary breath holding, he may become slightly bluish in colour. Then breathing begins again and the casualty will make uncontrolled movements of the arms and/or legs. Twitching of the face and body may also occur. The uncontrolled movements will usually last for about 2–4 minutes, gradually becoming less violent. The casualty regains consciousness shortly after the twitching movements cease. Fits may, however, vary in severity and duration. Very slight fits may occur with momentary loss of consciousness and very little movement.

After the fit, the casualty will have a loss of memory, but memory will return. The extent of loss of memory for recent events is a useful rough guide to the severity of the fit, in a similar way to the loss of memory following concussion (page 69).

Very severe burns can occur in people who have an epileptic attack near open fires. Here is an added reason to guard all open fires and other such dangers.

TREATMENT

Any casualty who is thought to be having a fit, convulsion or epileptic attack should be placed in the unconscious position. Hard objects should be moved away from the casualty in case an uncontrolled movement of a limb results in a blow or bang, thus causing further injury. *Gentle* restraint to prevent damage and cut down movement may be used, but forcible restraint to stop movement *must not* be applied.

When the casualty regains consciousness, he will usually appear dazed and will not remember what happened to him, so keep him quiet and at rest.

All casualties who have been unconscious must be seen by a doctor, so send them to hospital.

If you think that a fit is due to a recent head injury, you must waste no time in getting the casualty to hospital as the fit may be due in this case to bleeding inside the skull (page 75).

Babies and young children who have epileptic attacks or convulsions must always be sent to hospital.

SUDDEN COLLAPSE

The medical and surgical treatment of the conditions which cause sudden collapse will obviously depend on the exact

TABLE 5.1

Injury	*Illness*
Sudden severe bleeding	Heart attack (coronary thrombosis)
Prolonged bleeding	Diabetes
Severe pain	Stroke (cerebral haemorrhage)
Chest injury	Allergy (anaphylaxis)
Spinal injury	Peritonitis
Extensive burns	Emotional upsets
Poisoning, including alcohol	Internal bleeding
Gassing	from a duodenal ulcer
Extensive injuries	from an ectopic pregnancy
	Food poisoning or illness associated
	with diarrhoea and vomiting
	Chilling (hypothermia)
	Heat exhaustion
	Perforated peptic ulcer (gastric or
	duodenal)

diagnosis of the cause of collapse. But, before looking in detail for causes of collapse, if

— the heart is not beating
— the casualty is not breathing
— the casualty is bleeding
— the casualty is unconscious

apply appropriate treatment.

Next, try to get some idea of why the casualty has collapsed.

The list (Table 5.1) is by no means complete, but gives some of the more common causes of sudden collapse following injury or illness.

Try to apply appropriate first-aid if you know what is the matter. If you do not know—or are not sure what is wrong —send the casualty to hospital so that the doctors there can apply treatment. Remember too the old adage that 'more is missed by not looking than by not knowing'.

MENTAL ILLNESS

MEDICAL INFORMATION

Only mental illness of sudden origin, or a serious breakdown of existing mental illness, are likely to present first-aid problems. Some people when mentally ill may show a pattern of behaviour which is only slightly different from their normal, but in others, behaviour may be so bizarre that this behaviour could be recognized as abnormal by anyone meeting that person for the first time.

When people behave in unusual ways, we have to accept that the person has reason for this unusual behaviour. The casualty, the first-aider, or both, may or may not understand why the behaviour is different, but if help has to be given, *the first-aider must begin by accepting the behaviour, whatever it is, and the casualty's need to behave in that way.*

Sometimes the reason for abnormal behaviour will be obvious—for example, following a life-threatening experience or a sudden bereavement. But in many cases the reason(s) for the change in the casualty's behaviour will not be obvious, nor indeed is it a first-aid problem to try to find out the reason(s). No amateur psychotherapy should be attempted! Leave this to the expert psychiatrist.

FIRST-AID for MENTALLY DISTURBED CASUALTIES

Approach the casualty calmly. Be natural and friendly towards anyone who appears to be behaving oddly. Ask them how they feel, what they believe to be the trouble and so on. In spite of the popular belief that mentally ill people are often dangerous, it is only very rarely that they become violent or aggressive—so, do not be afraid.

Comfort, kindliness, friendliness and a willingness to listen sympathetically will help in nearly every case. Mentally ill people are sick people and require compassion, acceptance and understanding to a greater extent than physically sick or injured people.

If people behave peculiarly and you think that they may be mentally ill, do not leave them alone in case they harm themselves. People who threaten suicide MUST NOT be left alone in case they carry out their threat. Particular care must be taken to escort such people even to the toilet, leaving the door ajar, to keep them away from upstairs windows, and away from medicines and poisons of all kinds. Always seek help at once from a doctor in such cases.

Casualties who are mentally ill need expert help. Call the doctor, therefore, as soon as you recognize that someone is mentally ill, or arrange for the casualty to be taken to hospital.

If you think that a person is mentally ill but he is unwilling to be helped, or is becoming a danger to himself or to other people, it may be necessary to inform the police as well as a doctor in order to deal effectively with the situation. Do not argue with the casualty—this will accomplish nothing useful.

People cannot be taken to hospital against their will unless certain legal formalities are accomplished. The doctor and the police both know how to deal with this situation, should it be necessary for the safety and well-being of the casualty or that of the community. Always seek help and try to remain on friendly terms with the casualty until help arrives.

MOTION SICKNESS

MEDICAL INFORMATION

Motion sickness is a general term used to describe nausea and sickness caused by the effects of movement of the body during travel, whether by car, air or sea, or even fairground amusement rides.

The sufferer from motion sickness usually experiences a feeling as if he is going to vomit—nausea—and may then become worse and actually begin vomiting. In severe cases, dizziness and continued vomiting may lead to quite severe general collapse.

HOW TO PREVENT MOTION SICKNESS

The first essential in prevention is to recognize that motion sickness may occur—this means that we have to foresee the kind of motion and the length of time during which the motion is likely to be experienced. Likely sufferers will also need to be identified.

With this information, these likely sufferers can be given a suitable dose of a motion sickness inhibitor and can then be given subsequent doses at intervals, if the journey is prolonged.

Motion sickness remedies are almost useless in the presence of vomiting—they require to be given in ample time, *before* the possible onset of the condition, in other words before the journey starts.

191

Many people who suffer from motion sickness are able to undertake journeys very successfully with the aid of drugs, properly administered. However, some unfortunates seem to be sick in spite of all the treatment mentioned here.

Drugs for the prevention of motion sickness should not be given to pregnant women or to car drivers.

HOW TO TREAT MOTION SICKNESS

The most obvious helpful measure is to stop travelling, if possible, as soon as nausea appears.

If, however, this is not practicable, as is the case on a ship, the sufferer should be given a suitable dose of motion sickness remedy in the hope that some of it may be absorbed and not lost with the next bout of vomiting, and will thus begin to help. He should then be put lying down, or in a position of rest if he cannot lie down. Rest and assurance that the journey will soon end are often helpful.

In prolonged sea voyages, very susceptible persons can become quite ill due to long continued sea-sickness. In repeated vomiting, much fluid is lost to the body, and efforts should be made to replace as much as possible by encouraging drinking. This should be given in sips to prevent stimulation of further vomiting. Medical aid should be sought, if possible, in these cases and where medical aid is available, the use of promethazine hydrochloride (Phenergan) by intramuscular injection in a dose of 50 mg for an adult is recommended. Children can be treated safely in the same manner with a proportionate dosage. Promethazine is also effective by mouth. Cure rates of 95 per cent are reported.

ABDOMINAL PAIN

MEDICAL INFORMATION

Abdominal pain can be of two main kinds.

(*i*) *Sharp stabbing or pricking pain*—usually made worse by moving, by pressure, by coughing and by sneezing. This kind of pain is found at a particular spot and is usually a more serious type of pain than colicky pain.

(*ii*) *Colicky pain*—a pain which comes and goes at intervals of about 2 or 3 minutes, and is not felt at a particular spot but over an area. Colicky pains are commonly felt around the middle region of the abdomen centred round and often just above the navel.

Both kinds of pain may occur together or separately. The pain may be accompanied by vomiting or diarrhoea or by general collapse. Fortunately, it is not the task of the first-aider to sort out the different causes of abdominal pain such as acute appendicitis, perforated duodenal ulcers, or pain associated with gastro-enteritis.

TREATMENT

Any abdominal pain which is more than transient and slight is an indication that the casualty should be seen by a doctor. Children, especially, who have abdominal pain which is other than transient or slight should always be seen by a doctor.

Casualties who complain of abdominal pain should be put at rest lying down and should be given nothing by mouth until seen by a doctor. Often such casualties will be more comfortable sitting up slightly with their knees bent, particularly if pain is severe. Encourage them to adopt the position which gives greatest relief. Any casualty having severe abdominal pain, particularly if the pain is sharp and the casualty looks ill or is collapsed, should be sent at once to hospital.

NEVER give laxatives or opening medicines to any casualty who complains of abdominal pain.

DIARRHOEA AND VOMITING

MEDICAL INFORMATION

Diarrhoea and vomiting of sudden origin may present as a first-aid problem. Often the cause is 'food poisoning'. Food poisoning rarely may be due to actual chemical poisoning of food, but is more commonly due to eating food contaminated by germs.

The casualty is often away from home when this illness afflicts him. The illness may begin with vomiting or with diarrhoea, but in the more severe forms of the illness, vomiting usually appears first, closely followed by diarrhoea. In severe cases, the casualty may be generally affected and feel weak, ill and collapsed. In less severe episodes, the casualty may feel fairly normal between the actual bouts of vomiting or diarrhoea. Colicky abdominal pains often accompany the condition. Fever may also be present. From an early stage of the illness and as a result of vomiting and diarrhoea, the casualty loses a lot of body fluid. He will thus become dehydrated soon if this fluid loss is not replaced.

FIRST-AID for DIARRHOEA AND VOMITING

Put the casualty to bed and arrange for a doctor to come and see the casualty. If general prostration is severe, however, send the casualty to hospital. Give nothing to eat.

The most important part of treatment is to try to replace the fluid loss by giving frequent small amounts of water, or other bland fluid, by mouth. Large amounts will cause vomiting. About half a cupful every 10–15 minutes for adults will be as much as can be managed usually. Children will require less. Children and adults will often accept and prefer fizzy drinks. The first-aider can be of great help by starting the treatment as soon as possible.

Always keep any suspect food or drink for bacteriological examination, making sure that no-one else can or will eat the food. Wash your own hands very thoroughly after touching any suspect food or after dealing with any diarrhoea or vomit. Similarly, keep any sample of vomit or diarrhoea, for bacteriological examination.

HERNIA

MEDICAL INFORMATION

A hernia (rupture) appears as a swelling, usually in the groin, but sometimes around the navel or as a bulge in an operation scar on the abdomen or groin. Due to a weakness in the abdominal wall, the gut or other abdominal content comes to lie under the skin instead of under the full thickness of the abdominal wall.

The lump may appear suddenly after exertion or coughing, or it may appear gradually. Unless the appearance of the swelling is very rapid or there is obstruction of the bowel associated with the hernia, the condition is usually painless.

TREATMENT

All new hernias and suspected hernias should be seen by a doctor, or sent to hospital. Until then, if at home, the casualty should be placed in bed with the knees drawn up and pillows under the thighs for support. The head and shoulders should be well supported on two or three pillows. This helps to relax the abdominal muscles and makes the casualty more comfortable.

If pain is colicky (page 193) or severe, or there is any inclination to feel sick or to vomit, the doctor should be told this when being asked to call, since these symptoms may mean obstruction of the bowel. If a doctor is not available, send the casualty to hospital.

PROTRUDING PILES

MEDICAL INFORMATION

Piles (haemorrhoids) are varicose veins at or near the anus. Occasionally, after the bowels have opened or following heavy work, the piles may protrude and be visible through the anus. The anus may then tighten round the base of the protruding veins and further increase the swelling.

TREATMENT

Bed rest and an ice pack or cold compresses applied to the affected region whilst lying face down in bed relieves pain and may allow sufficient shrinkage to occur for the piles to return to their original site.

A doctor should be asked to see the casualty, and until then the casualty should be kept face down in bed with the ice pack or cold compresses over the affected area.

OTHER MEDICAL CONDITIONS
POISONING

Most cases of poisoning are *easily preventable*. Every opportunity should therefore be taken to try to educate people in the safe handling of poisonous materials of all kinds. Storage, methods of use and precautions to be followed should be printed clearly on labels and all instructions should be read and followed by the user.

Many cases of poisoning occur at home to children—so, lock medicine cabinets and discard half-used and old medicines. Keep household cleaners out of reach of toddlers. Poisoning is easy to prevent, but it can present considerable difficulties in treatment.

ROUTES OF ENTRY OF POISONS INTO THE BODY

Poisons can get into the body by three main routes:

(*i*) by mouth,
(*ii*) by inhalation or
(*iii*) through the skin.

With some poisons a combination of methods of entry may apply.

First-aid will vary in each case, according to the poison and the route of entry. Variation will also occur if the casualty is conscious or unconscious, and if there is any specific first-aid for that particular poison.

The first-aid for poisoning by mouth

1. ACT QUICKLY—and calmly.
   ↓
2. **If Unconscious**
   TREAT AS AN UNCONSCIOUS
   CASUALTY— Place the casualty in the unconscious position with a slight head down tip and send to hospital quickly, together with any clues as to what the poison might be, such as tablets, empty bottles, syringes, vomited materials and so on.
   ↓
3. **If Conscious**—Send quickly to hospital. Try to determine the nature of the poison by asking the casualty what he took in case he becomes unconscious.
   ↓
   DO NOT make
   the casualty
   vomit
   ↓
   DO NOT GIVE
   ANYTHING BY MOUTH
   ↓
4. NOW SEND QUICKLY—If conscious, send in the first available car.
   TO HOSPITAL   —If unconscious, send for an ambulance and tell them why.

ALWAYS SEND CLUES—Send empty bottles, tablets, vomited material, berries
TO HOSPITAL with   or anything else which may help the doctors in
the casualty   hospital to identify the poison and the dose.

Remember to use the first available transport if the casualty is conscious. Unconscious children can be taken to hospital in a car, in the unconscious position, lying on an adult's lap with a head-down tip.

First-aid for poisoning by inhalation

(1) Remove the casualty from the contaminated atmosphere. Make sure that rescuers do not become casualties. If there is enough poison to overcome one person, anyone who breathes that atmosphere may be similarly overcome.

(2) Check for breathing—if the casualty is not breathing, apply artificial respiration.

(3) If the casualty is unconscious, treat for unconsciousness in the usual way.

(4) If the casualty is conscious and has difficulty in breathing, place him in one of the positions shown in *Figure 5.1*, which ease breathing, and send him to hospital in this position.

First-aid for poisoning through the skin

(1) Remove the casualty from any obvious pool of con-contamination and check for breathing. If the casualty is not breathing, apply artificial respiration.

(2) If the casualty is unconscious, place him in the unconscious position and treat as usual for unconsciousness.

(3) As quickly as you can, remove any chemical from the skin by washing, by removal of contaminated clothing, and by further washing. If many helpers are present, this step may be taken at the same time as the casualty is being given artificial respiration, or while he is being treated for unconsciousness. The aim is to get rid of any further chemical from the skin and thus prevent further poisoning. Flush the chemical from the skin with large amounts of water.

Take care that rescuers do not become contaminated and so become casualties.

POISON INFORMATION CENTRES

Poison information centres exist to give information about poisonous substances and to advise on the treatment of poisoning.

We suggest that readers may wish to list the telephone number of their nearest poison information centre in the following space *and* beside their telephone.

PESTICIDES

Like any other poisonous substances, pesticides should be handled with care. The instructions on the manufacturer's label should be carefully studied and followed. This will *prevent* poisoning.

The most hazardous pesticides cannot be sold to amateur gardeners so that any cases of poisoning which occur are probably due either to gross misuse or to neglect of common-sense precautions—or to both.

Those who work in horticulture or agriculture may, however, be exposed to a wider variety of more active materials. If pesticide poisoning is suspected, the priorities will be to apply first-aid, to send for help and to find the container of the pesticide, which should state on it the nature of the active chemical and the appropriate first-aid. It is therefore important to locate the container, or any leaflet which went with the container, so that the *appropriate* first-aid is applied rather than some form of erratic action. As in any case of poisoning, send containers, leaflets and any other information to hospital with the casualty.

In addition, if chemical contamination of skin or eyes is present, the casualty should have the chemical washed out of the eyes and off the skin at once, and should have all contaminated clothing removed.

A few notes are given below about certain pesticides which present special first-aid problems.

Poisoning by dinitro compounds

Dinitro compounds are absorbed mainly through the skin. The casualty should therefore be treated as for chemical contamination—wash or shower with water and remove contaminated clothing.

After this, the casualty should be kept flat and *at rest*. On no account allow the casualty to walk or move himself. Keep him in a cool place and try to keep him cool prior to sending him to hospital.

Organophosphorus poisoning

Organophosphorus compounds are absorbed mainly through the skin. The casualty should therefore be treated as for chemical contamination—wash or shower with water and remove contaminated clothing.

Watch the casualty's breathing most carefully. *Breathing may suddenly stop.* Give artificial respiration at once if breathing ceases. Send for a doctor or for a nurse who can administer atropine by injection, if by this means atropine can be given more quickly than by sending the casualty at once to hospital.

Organophosphorus compounds cause poisoning by depressing the action of an enzyme, cholinesterase. The ideal treatment is to give a cholinesterase reactivator (pralidoxime. P 25) at the earliest possible moment. Supplies of pralidoxime are usually available only from hospital, and until the casualty can be taken to hospital, or the cholinesterase reactivator to the casualty, *atropine sulphate should be given*. In advanced first-aid, atropine sulphate will usually be the only drug available unless the emergency has been foreseen and pralidoxime is available.

Atropine should be given in a *dose of 1–4 mg every hour intravenously* if necessary. In mild cases of poisoning, this may be enough to relieve the symptoms. However, if prompt improvement does not occur, or if deterioration begins, further doses of atropine should be given. If the casualty has not responded to 10 mg of atropine, the use of a cholinesterase reactivator is a matter of urgency.

Under no circumstances should atropine injections be delayed until cholinesterase reactivators such as pralidoxime are available. Atropine should be given in amounts which cause dilated pupils, dry mouth and raised heart rate, and may have to be given for 24–48 hours.

Cholinesterase reactivator should be given intramuscularly or intravenously as early as possible and preferably at the same time as atropine.

Breathing must be watched carefully during transfer to hospital, and thereafter. Use a sucker if necessary to clear the airways. Morphine *must not* be given.

TETANUS PREVENTION

Tetanus toxoid given by injection *before* any injury happens is the method of choice in preventing tetanus. First-aiders should therefore take any opportunity which presents to encourage people to have these protective inoculations, and to make sure that they are, themselves, suitably immunized.

Tetanus ('lockjaw') is a disease which can follow cuts or wounds of any kind. It is a preventable disease, and should therefore be prevented.

SNAKEBITE

MEDICAL INFORMATION

Reid, writing about snakebite in the tropics has this to say: 'The paramount fact about bites of man by poisonous snakes is that more than one-half of the victims will have minimal or no poisoning. Only about one-quarter will develop systemic poisoning. Hence poisonous snakebite is not synonymous with snakebite poisoning.' With snakebite, as in other situations, the principle of the calculated risk is applied. Although it might be advisable to vary the treatment according to the country, the kind of casualty, the availability of help from people near at hand, the kind of snake, the site of the bite, the equipment available and so on, the inclusion of such variables would result in recommendations which would be impossibly confusing. Clear, simple advice is therefore preferable to a set of complicated instructions.

TREATMENT

The first-aid for snakebite occurring anywhere in the world is to

leave the bite alone and go quickly to the nearest hospital (self-help)

or

take the casualty at once to the nearest hospital (first-help).

A wound dressing should be applied to the bite to prevent any further contamination or infection, following the general principles of wound treatment.

If possible send a message to the hospital to say that a casualty who has been bitten by a snake—naming the kind of snake—will be arriving at a certain time.

A few additional points may be helpful.

—A casualty who *thinks* he has been bitten by a snake, or who has been *half-bitten,* that is, bitten without venom injection, or more *deeply bitten* by a snake—whether poisonous or non-poisonous—is usually suffering from *fright and fear of rapid death.*

—The danger of poisonous snake bites have been greatly exaggerated, so reassure the casualty at once that he is unlikely to die. Any casualty who has only been *half-bitten,* even by a known poisonous snake such as a cobra, viper or sea snake, will develop no significant poisoning because little or no venom is injected. Reid has stated that at least half of the casualties bitten by poisonous snakes have no venom injected, that is, half of the casualties are only half-bitten.

> *If adequate medical treatment is received within a few hours of a bite, serious poisoning is rare and death is exceptional.*

—The bitten part should, if possible, be kept at rest, but not at the expense of delaying arrival in hospital. For example, it is better to walk on a leg which is bitten and get to hospital soon, rather than wait to be carried and thus delay arrival at hospital. Panic running, of course, should be avoided, as the increase in circulation resulting from running may increase the rate of absorption of poison from the bite, especially if the bite is in the leg.

—In Great Britain, the adder *(vipera berus)* is the only poisonous snake. The dangers of this snake have been very greatly exaggerated.

—If the snake is dead or can be killed by some blows *behind* the head, it should be taken to hospital to aid identification and thus help to decide appropriate treatment. Handle dead snakes by the tail only, and with care! The reason for using blows *behind* the head is that the appearance of the head is usually the main means of identifying a snake.

A word about prevention may be approprate. Most snake bites occur in daylight and on the feet and legs because the casualty treads on or near a snake. In country where dangerous snakes are known to exist, boots are advisable. At night, a torch should be used.

footnote to snakebite

Lest there be any misunderstanding about this section, we should like to remind the reader that the advice given is for the *first-aid*—not the definitive treatment of snakebite.

In the past, the recommended first-aid treatment for snakebite tended to be rather dramatic, but today such heroic treatment is not recommended.

CHAPTER 6

EMERGENCY CHILDBIRTH

Our birth is but a sleep and a forgetting.
WILLIAM WORDSWORTH

FIRST-AID IN EMERGENCY CHILDBIRTH

Under normal conditions the management of childbirth is outside the scope of first-aid. Only if it is COMPLETELY IMPOSSIBLE to obtain skilled professional help will a first-aider take charge.

MEDICAL INFORMATION

Childbirth (labour) can be described in three stages.
  (1) Regular labour pains occur, and later become stronger. The interval between the pains gets shorter.
  (2) The child is born.
  (3) The placenta (afterbirth) is expelled.

THE FIRST STAGE

By regular contractions, the muscle of the uterus (womb) causes the cervix (neck) of the uterus to open. From being a tightly closed muscular ring, it must dilate (enlarge) to allow the passage of the baby *(Figures 6.1 and 6.2)*.

During the later stages of pregnancy the muscle of the uterus contracts and becomes firm. These contractions are painless and often pass unnoticed. The onset of labour is

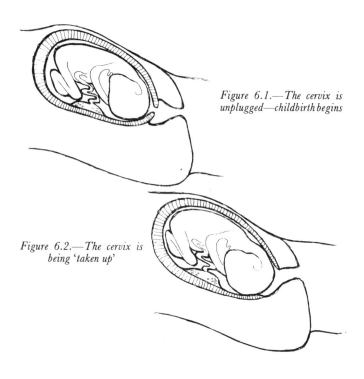

Figure 6.1.—The cervix is unplugged—childbirth begins

Figure 6.2.—The cervix is being 'taken up'

marked by these contractions becoming more powerful and occurring at regular intervals. These regular contractions are called *labour pains*. The mother notices them first in the lower abdomen and they are often associated with backache. During this stage of labour the membranes around the baby usually burst, and some fluid leaves the uterus and may wet the floor or bed. This is often called 'the breaking of the waters'. Before this happens, at the beginning of labour, a little blood or slime is sometimes passed from the vagina. This is normal, and is due to unplugging of the cervix.

THE SECOND STAGE

The uterine contractions become stronger and cause the head and body of the baby to pass down the birth canal. The mother tends to bear down and to hold her breath with each contraction.

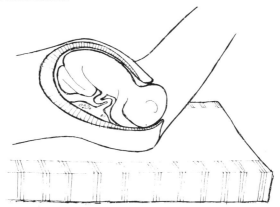

Figure 6.3.—The head is 'crowned' by the outlet

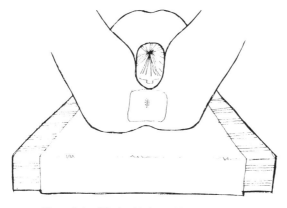

Figure 6.4.—The head is born. Note pad over anus

207

Just before the head appears at the outlet a fullness can be seen behind the birth canal and the rectal contents may be forced out. Soon after this, the baby's hair appears followed by more and more of the head with each contraction. The head is then born, usually with the baby facing backwards *(Figures 6.3 and 6.4)*. Often the head is seen to rotate *(Figure 6.5)* before the shoulders and body are born with a further contraction.

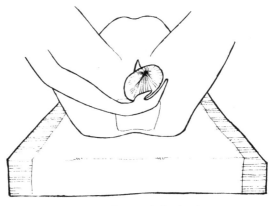

Figure 6.5.—Support the head as it rotates

There is now usually a flow of blood-stained fluid. The baby is still attached to the mother by the umbilical cord.

THE THIRD STAGE

After a pause of some 5–10 minutes the uterus undergoes further contractions to expel the placenta into the birth canal and out of the body. There may now be a further loss of blood.

EMERGENCY CHILDBIRTH

The AIMS of FIRST-AID for EMERGENCY CHILDBIRTH

—Make every endeavour to obtain the help of a doctor or midwife. A telephone call (the number is usually 999) will often bring the maternity 'flying squad' which exists to help with emergency maternity care.

—Take the expectant mother to hospital quickly, but without panic haste. There is often still time for the baby to be born in hospital.

However, if birth outside of hospital is inevitable,

—prevent infection of both mother and baby by scrupulous cleaning of the hands and by using clean linen, and

—care for the baby and mother after delivery.

PREPARATIONS FOR LABOUR

If it is impossible to send the expectant mother to a medical unit, she should be removed to a warm sheltered place and put into bed. Failing this a mattress or other makeshift bed should be arranged on the floor. Collect some clean linen and blankets for use by mother and baby.

THE FIRST-AID MANAGEMENT OF CHILDBIRTH

The first stage

During the early part of the first stage, the expectant mother should be encouraged to empty and to keep empty both her bladder and bowel. It is at this time of labour that the first-aider is on his mettle and all his basic training now counts. The patient is worried and often requires reassurance. It is for the first-aider, however apprehensive he may feel inwardly, to put on a bold front, to remain calm and to be obviously in control of the situation. This will be of immense value to the mother.

The second stage

In the later part of the first stage and the early part of the second stage, when the contractions are becoming stronger and closer together in time, place the mother in the un-conscious position. This is the most comfortable position, and is the same as the relaxed position used in ante-natal care.*

Take this opportunity to wash and scrub your hands—in running water if at all possible. When the contractions occur every 2–3 minutes and are more powerful, turn the mother on to her back so that she can pull on the backs of her thighs as the head is born. Encourage her to hold her breath and push with the uterine contractions. As soon as the head first appears, place a large sterile or clean pad over the anus. A field dressing or sanitary towel will do. Next, place a clean towel or sheet below her buttocks. As the head is being born, tell the mother to pant hard with the contraction. After the baby's head is born, it will rotate. The shoulders and body will then be born quite quickly. Gently support the baby's head and shoulders as it is being born *(Figure 6.6 and 6.7)*.

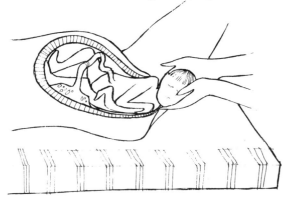

Figure 6.6.—Gently support the head as the shoulders are born. Do not pull

* Entonox (a mixture of nitrous oxide and oxygen) is available in many ambulances as a pain reliever. It can safely be used by *self-administration* to relieve the contraction pains felt by the mother in the second stage of labour.

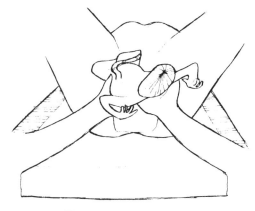

Figure 6.7.—The baby is born

Do not pull on the child or on the cord. Allow the mother to push the child out. When the baby is born, gently wipe any mucus from the baby's mouth and make sure it begins to breathe. If it does not breathe, hold it upside-down—being very careful that the rather slippery skin does not cause you to drop the baby—and allow any fluid to drain out of the mouth and nose *(Figure 6.8)*. While doing this, gently rub

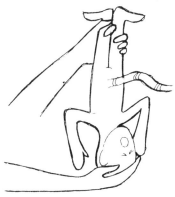

Figure 6.8.—Allow any fluid to drain from the baby's nose or mouth. Grip the legs firmly as shown

or pat the baby's back—this will often help breathing to
start. Artificial respiration is rarely needed, but if it is,
cover the baby's nose and mouth with your mouth and use
very gentle quick puffs only. When the baby is breathing
regularly the umbilical cord should be tied off twice on the
baby's side *(Figure 6.9)* and once on the mother's side. Firm

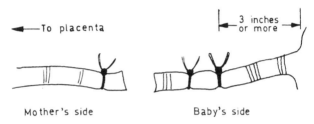

*Figure 6.9.—Tie the cord twice on the baby's side, once on the
mother's side*

knotting with string does well for this purpose. Leave a
minimum of 8 cm (3 inches) of cord on the baby's side when
cutting the cord. Tying and cutting the cord does not hurt
the baby or the mother. There is no *need* to tie and cut the cord.
It is convenient to separate the baby from the placenta by
cutting the cord (this often makes baby parking easier!) but
neither mother nor baby will come to any harm if the cord
is neither cut nor tied. If you are going to cut the cord you
should of course tie it first.

Now place the baby, front down, head to one side, on the
mother's abdomen, with the head down over one side. This
will keep the baby warm and will allow any fluid to drain
out of the airway. The mother will probably half sit up to
see the new baby. Tell her whether the baby is a boy or a
girl and reassure her that it is normal and healthy.

The third stage

During the third stage keep the mother covered with blankets but do not use hot water bottles even if she is shivering. The placenta should normally be delivered without discomfort within 20 minutes. DO NOT pull on the cord to hurry the delivery of the placenta. Always save the placenta for examination by the doctor or midwife *(Figure 6.10)*.

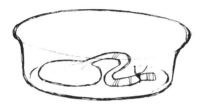

Figure 6.10.—Always keep the placenta

If the placenta is not delivered by about 20 minutes after the birth of the child, the first-aider should look for signs of internal bleeding which may be taking place *(see page 35)*.

THE BABY

By this time the baby will be crying regularly. This is normal and is the best way of getting the lungs properly inflated. Wrap the infant firmly in a clean sheet so that the limbs are folded to the body in the natural fashion. Give the baby to the mother to cuddle and nurse. This is satisfying to the mother and may stimulate the muscles of the uterus to contract firmly, thus preventing internal bleeding.

Incubators for babies

Newborn babies who are premature or of low birth weight —225 kg (under 5 lb) or less—may require to be placed in an incubator in order to conserve their body heat while being transferred to hospital. If the baby is born more than 2 months before the expected date, it is likely to be small. Such babies die very easily from cold. They should be placed in a room at 21–25°C (70–78°F) if possible, and should be kept away from draughts.

If the baby is small or premature, do not expose it to cold rooms or to the weather unless this is absolutely unavoidable. Small or premature babies are especially susceptible to cold. Arrange to transfer such babies to hospital in an incubator. (*See* page 168 for a description of chilling in babies.)

tail piece

The first-aider should carry out only the simplest assistance and hand over to a doctor or midwife at the earliest possible moment. Any first-aider finding himself acting as emergency midwife should take comfort in the fact that most deliveries are perfectly normal and require little assistance. His main usefulness will be to provide the one cool head in a highly emotional situation. Nature often does the rest!

CHAPTER 7

MISCELLANEOUS

THE EFFECTIVE FIRST-AIDER

Any person who gives first-aid must learn to conduct himself or herself in a calm, sympathetic and confident manner. This need is especially important in people qualified in advanced first-aid and who, by the nature of their work—nurses, medical students, ambulance attendants, and full-time first-aiders in industry, for example—are expected to conduct themselves in an expert manner.

Effective first-aid is much more than applying the first-aid treatment as laid down in the book. Such first-aid treatment can be given gently or roughly; calmly or in an excited manner; with regard for the feelings of the casualty or without; confidently or timidly. Control of one's self undoubtedly comes first, but control of others in emergency conditions is equally important. The effective first-aider will make sure that every incident is handled quietly, calmly and effectively, and that not only the casualties but also any other people in the area are dealt with competently and sympathetically. Handling of emergency situations in this way will ensure more help for injured people than can be accurately measured.

It may be appropriate here to include some remarks which are mainly for those whose job in first-aid is a full-time one.

(*i*) *Personal appearance* must be neat, clean and tidy. Uniform should be worn so that easy identification is possible—and the uniform must be kept neat and clean. A high level of personal hygiene is essential. The effect on a casualty of a person in unkempt clothing with dirty hands and finger

215

nails offering to deal with his wound can be imagined . . . .
Wound infection can best be kept to a minimum by good
treatment techniques and by scrupulous personal hygiene.

(ii) *Telling the casualty* what is the matter and how he is
likely to progress is one of the very difficult problems which
may face people who carry out emergency or first-aid
treatment—including doctors, nurses and first-aiders. Saying
nothing will increase fear and anxiety, but saying too much
can cause needless alarm and despondency. Some casualties
will want to know exactly what is the matter, others will not.
Following injury, some casualties may be very upset emo-
tionally, while others may be calm.

The only way to deal with these problems is to try to
assess the needs of each individual casualty, and to try to
deal with these needs as sympathetically as you can. It is,
however, always unwise to give direct replies to questions
about the extent of the injuries and the time required for
full recovery. No satisfactory answer to these questions is
possible until a full hospital assessment has been made. If
the casualty insists on discussing his injuries with you, try to
reassure him that the doctors in hospital will be able to
help him and that he should recover.

(iii) *Actions* speak louder than words is an old adage but
especially true in first-aid. Practice in simulated emergencies
will help towards producing good, calm, smooth and un-
hurried action when a real emergency is faced.

(iv) *Tone of voice* conveys almost as much as what is said
to any listener. Shouting implies excitement—and excitement will be conveyed to the casualty if you shout. Try to
give any instructions, requests or information in a calm and
soothing tone of voice, thus letting the casualty know that he
is in good hands and that the person dealing with him is
unflustered.

(v) *Giving information to relatives* may often be a problem.
In general, it is better initially to say too little than too
much. It is also better to admit ignorance than to give bad

or misleading information. The public have a right to expect *intelligent* and *informed* opinions about the casualty. If you cannot give such information, refrain from giving any; wild and uninformed guesses merely create further distress for relatives and more problems for doctors.

It is nearly always difficult to do worth while things—and practice is often a prerequisite of success. The control of oneself, the acquisition of knowledge of first-aid and the practice necessary to keep that knowledge in good operating condition are all part of that professionalism which distinguishes the expert in this, as in any other field. Make sure that you are classed with the professionals, by attention to the points which are contained in this section.

DEALING WITH CHILDREN, TODDLERS AND INFANTS

Approximately one-quarter of the casualties attending hospital accident and emergency departments are children. Similarly, at home, many of the occasions which give rise to a need for first-aid may be connected with children.

It is therefore most useful to know something of the best ways of dealing with children, and to realize that, in order to administer good first-aid, it is essential that you make sure that the child is not frightened, but has confidence in you. The approach to the child can determine whether as a first-aider you will be accepted or rejected. This acceptance or rejection by the child will make the subsequent task easy or, in cases of rejection, may make good work almost impossible.

A child's reaction to injury will depend on a number of factors, such as age, the amount of pain, and the child's ability to express what he or she feels to be wrong. A few ideas are given below on how to approach and manage children or toddlers who are injured.

—Always approach the child through the mother, father, guardian, elder brother or sister. Speak *first* to the mother or to the people whom the child already knows and trusts. Let the child see that the mother trusts you, and that she expects you to help. Ask the mother what has happened and what the child—using his or her name if possible—did to sustain the injury. *Then, and only then,* when you are sure that the child has had a good look at you and accepts you, should you begin to speak to the child. If you do not meet with acceptance, ask any further questions through the mother until the child does accept you. A child's reaction to almost anything tends to be of the all or nothing kind. For example, the child will either accept or reject you. A middle course is unusual. Try to make sure in your early dealings with the child that you are accepted—it makes everything else so much easier!

—If the child's mother or guardian is frightened, try to calm the mother or guardian. Their fears will be transmitted to the child. If this fear is relieved, it will be reflected in the behaviour of the child who trusts them.

—A child is dependent. He or she needs somebody's hand to hold, and somebody to look to for comfort and reassurance. Never separate the child from this person.

—A child copes less well with fright and pain than an adult so try to avoid doing or saying anything which will give rise to fright or pain.

—Toddlers do not take kindly to restraint. Attempts to restrain them will probably lead to scenes, and to rejection of the person who tries to inflict the restraint.

—Infants cannot tell you what is the matter so try to find this out from the mother. Slightly older children may be short of words and find difficulty in expressing what they feel to be wrong with them. Try to help by suggesting words for them to choose—but always give them a choice so that you do not suggest what they should say!

—Although children may be short of words, they are logical and will usually cooperate well if they understand what has to be done and why. Explanations should *always* be given of what you are doing or going to do. Explain through the mother if the child is very young, but try to keep the child's confidence by telling him what you are going to do. Silence can be terrifying to an infant and to an older child—so keep talking about what you are doing or will do, and gain the child's cooperation. If what you have to do will be painful, say so *before* you do it, and say why you have to do it. Lack of explanations can lead to a child seeing a stretcher and thinking that it is a coffin. It is not hard to imagine how such a child may feel and behave on seeing the stretcher!

—Children do not malinger. If a child looks ill or complains of pain, always take this at face value and act accordingly.

—Try to spare children from horrid sights so that first-aid leaves no mental scars.

OBSERVATION OF THE CASUALTY

The job of the first-aider is not completed when a casualty has been correctly diagnosed and treated. A further task remains—to continue observation and treatment until the casualty is handed over to a doctor, to skilled ambulance men, or to the hospital staff.

Situations can change; the condition of the casualty can improve or deteriorate and these differences must be observed so that appropriate action can be taken. Careful observation is particularly important in the case of casualties who cannot do things for themselves or who are unconscious.

Observations can be of two kinds:

—those which necessitate action being taken and

—those which record the state of events at a particular point in time and can be used to build a progress record.

OBSERVATIONS WHICH NECESSITATE ACTION

It is obviously important to make observations so that appropriate action can be taken; for example, to recognize that a casualty is becoming unconscious, very restless or is starting to bleed.

OTHER OBSERVATIONS

It is often equally important, in order to help the doctors in hospital, to make observations AND TO RECORD the state of events at a particular point in time. For example, a pulse rate which rises as time passes cannot be assessed quickly, easily or with certainty unless the pulse rate and the time are written down regularly. Similarly, if the observer changes from a first-aider at the scene of an incident, to an ambulance attendant *en route* for hospital, to a nursing sister and finally to a doctor in hospital, little can be learned with certainty unless observations are made properly *and* written down and passed on.

The pulse

At each contraction of the heart a surge of blood is forced into the aorta—the large artery connected to the heart—and the recoil of this thrust of blood is continued as a pulsation through all the arteries of the body. The pulse can therefore be felt in any artery which is sufficiently near the surface; the most convenient is the radial artery, which runs down the thumb side of the front of the wrist on the outer side of the tendon.

To take the pulse, place your index, middle and ring fingers on the front of the wrist along the course of the artery. Support the back of the wrist with your thumb, and gently press the artery against the underlying bone. The beat of the artery, which is called the pulse, will now be felt.

The following characteristics should be noted:

Rate—recorded as the number of beats per minute. taken over at least half a minute.

Strength—full, weak, or imperceptible.

Rhythm—regular or irregular.

The average adult pulse rate is about 75, but normal pulses vary between 60 and 90.

What to look for and record

Having made an initial assessment of the casualty and some brief notes of the condition(s) found and the time, the need is then to record simple data about the general condition and in particular cases to note any *changes* for better or for worse which occur.

New complaints by the casualty should be noted and if the reason for any change is known, it should be recorded. It is particularly important in casualties who have suffered a head injury to record as fully as possible what was observed about the level of consciousness at first and then at further intervals of time, and also to note the pulse rate (*see* page 53).

Specific examples of the need for observation are given in the text but the general need for good observation and records cannot be overemphasized. Observations are of little value if they are not acted upon or communicated.

Tables 7.1 and 7.2 give specimens of forms which may be of use to first-aiders in making notes. These types of notes should always be sent with the casualty to hospital.

NEW ADVANCED FIRST-AID

TABLE 7.1

INITIAL ASSESSMENT REPORT

Casualty's name
       address
       telephone number

Employer's name
       address
       telephone number

Next of kin's name
       address
       telephone number

    Has next of kin been told?   Yes ☐
                                    No ☐

- -

What happened (briefly)?

How did it happen?

Injuries/illness diagnosed?

What treatment given?

Disposal   hospital ☐
             home   ☐
             work   ☐

Signed......................................

Date...................................

222

TABLE 2

PROGRESS REPORT

Record data about

—general condition	Improving? Worsening?
—conscious/unconscious	Improving? Worsening?
—pain	Where? Why?
—colour	Flushed, pink, pale, blue and so on
—complaints by the casualty	Pain, feeling sick, dizzy and so on

ALWAYS RECORD THE TIME of any OBSERVATION

Time	*Report or observation*

Signed...

Date...

RECORDS

Records are the documents, or even scraps of paper, on which information is written down. Information which is written down can then be

—passed on to other people,
—used by other people,
—used to recall events against a time scale, and
—kept for future reference.

In all medical work, including first-aid and the treatment of minor injuries, there is a need to produce good written records of the events which have occurred and the treatment which has been carried out. We have already referred to the extreme importance of good notes and have emphasized the need to record the pulse rate against time in the section on bleeding. These are obvious examples of a general need for records.

In carrying out the full treatment of minor injuries, particularly in an industrial or office context, there is also a need to produce good records of what injury was sustained, of how the injury was said to have occurred, of the treatment carried out and of whether the casualty resumed full or restricted work. or was sent home or to hospital.

The importance of making good notes at the time is that this will greatly assist doctors and others, who see the casualty after the first-aider, to carry out speedy and appropriate treatment. Good notes made at the time can also protect the first-aider against allegations of faulty or inadequate first-aid if the notes show clearly that good first-aid was in fact carried out.

Therefore, *always make good notes at the time,* and hand over some written information whenever you pass on a casualty for further treatment.

TRANSPORTING CASUALTIES—SOME APHORISMS

Bleeding casualties travel badly. However, a short smooth

journey early may be better than delaying, resuscitating and then travelling.

Leg elevation and a head-down tip can be a life-saving measure for any casualty who has bled a lot. Such simple measures are not used in many cases where their application could greatly benefit the casualty.

Burned casualties travel well in the first 2 hours, and less well after this due to fluid loss from the circulation.

An ambulance is not always the best transport—the first available suitable vehicle may get the casualty to hospital much sooner, and may thus be better.

INDUSTRIAL FIRST-AID

Industries vary widely in character and therefore in their needs for rescue, first-aid and the treatment of minor injuries. Good industrial first-aid in any particular situation is nothing more than good first-aid applied to the special needs of that situation. The principles of first-aid as self-help or as first-help apply in exactly the same way to industrial first-aid as to any other situation in which general or special problems may present.

The need for rescue may present highly specialized problems. This is dealt with on pages 245 *et seq*.

In industry, the treatment of minor injuries will depend upon the skill of the first-aider in discriminating those injuries which he should or should not treat, and on the further on-the-spot help, including supervision, which is afforded. No precise rules can be laid down about what should be done, but at all times the interests of the casualty are paramount. No first-aider should attempt definitive treatment of any injury unless he is *absolutely* sure that he is competent to do so.

In summary, therefore, there is no special subject of industrial first-aid which is different in essence from good first-aid. Industrial first-aid is first-aid applied to special needs. The efficient treatment of minor injuries after good discrimination, and knowledge of emergency procedures and perhaps of rescue, are additional common requirements. Incidents in industry may be of a special kind due to the hazards or process involved, and the incidents may at times involve multiple casualties. However, the principles of good first-aid still apply.

REAGENT IMPREGNATED STRIPS

Reagent impregnated strips may be useful in ambulances or first-aid centres to determine rapidly such things as the presence of glucose or blood in urine, and the blood glucose level. Instructions for use are given on the packets.

The strips should be used by people who are familiar with their use—usually a doctor or nurse. It is worth keeping a packet of these strips in places where a doctor or nurse may be asked to see a casualty, in view of the rapid information which the strips can give.

Test	Strip
Glucose in urine	Labstix (or Clinistix)
Blood in urine	Labstix (or Hemastix)
Blood glucose level	Dextrostix

THE TREATMENT OF MINOR INJURIES

DISCRIMINATION

The first problem in treating minor injuries is to decide which injuries are in fact minor, and can or should be treated by non-medically trained or qualified personnel. Unfortunately, there is no easy guide line which can be laid down, except to say that if any shadow of doubt crosses the first-aider's mind about the exact nature or situation of the injury, or about the correct treatment of the injury, then the casualty must be passed on at once to a hospital or to a doctor. Never give definitive treatment for something you are not sure about; give first-aid and pass the casualty on. Doctors always prefer to see and to advise on the correct treatment of injuries shortly after the injury has occurred, rather than to clear up messes or to sort out the results of inadequate or less skilled treatment at a later date.

Anyone who attempts definitive treatment of other than obviously trivial skin grazes must avoid such pitfalls as incised wounds of fingers and wrist *with* underlying tendon or nerve injury, punctured wounds of the groin, crutch and buttocks with damage to arteries and abdominal contents, and foreign bodies IN the eye with no obvious wound of entry. Many other examples could be given. The rule, however, is simple: if in doubt, pass the casualty on to a more experienced person. Practise being suspicious and doubtful about the full extent of any injury.

The casualty's interests are served best by a cautious approach as to what to treat, and by a readiness to seek further advice. This applies equally to doctors as to first-aiders!

Table 7.3 is a list of conditions which may appear simple and are not, and should always be seen by a doctor after first-aid has been given.

TABLE 7.3

A danger list of conditions which should not be treated definitively as minor injuries even though they appear to be minor
Unconsciousness, for however short a time
Suspected internal bleeding. Internal bleeding may arise with little damage externally—from blast injuries, stab wounds and crushing injuries
Stab wounds or punctured wounds. Be specially careful of wounds in the neck, chest, abdomen, loin and groin areas
Wounds near joints. These may penetrate into the joint
Blunt injury to the eye and black eyes
Possible fractures. Many 'sprains' turn out to be fractures. An X-ray (radiograph) is the only sure way of knowing

MINOR TREATMENT

Steri-strip skin closures are an effective and painless way of taping skin edges together. This method of skin closure has superseded the stitching of minor wounds in many cases. It gives excellent cosmetic results, is painless, and the casualty likes the method. The end appearance of this method of skin closure is often better than can be achieved by stitching, and Steri-strip closure is a much more convenient procedure. It is especially suitable for children.

FIRST-AID IN ROAD INJURIES

Because the management of roadside incidents and the treatment of casualties arising from them are, unfortunately, such common problems, we have gathered together into one section a discussion about some of the dangers and difficulties, even though some of the material already appears elsewhere in the book.

In many countries, road injuries are amongst the principal causes of death, disability and hospitalization. Road injuries represent an enormous need both for preventive activity and for good first-aid. When injuries have occurred good first-aid can save lives, can help to minimize the pain and suffering and can prevent injuries from getting worse.

Good first-aid for road casualties is based on the same principles as good first-aid for any casualty anywhere. With road injury casualties, however, there may be a few special factors worth mentioning.

SAFETY AT THE SCENE OF THE INCIDENT

Do not become the next casualty. If you are on a road where fast traffic is flowing and you find a casualty in the middle of the road, try to send two people—one in each direction—to signal to the traffic to slow down. You should not, of course, move any casualty unless he is in a position of immediate danger until you have examined him and dealt with his injuries. If you have to venture out into a road at night, try to wear something white or conspicuous. See that other people who help do the same thing and are aware of the hazards.

At night, this warning is especially important, otherwise a small incident can become a disastrous and multiple fatal one. Make sure that you do not stand between a damaged or parked car and oncoming or passing traffic.

Switch off the lights and the ignition of all crashed vehicles. This will lessen the fire risk and may prevent carbon monoxide poisoning or possible further injury from moving parts.

No smoking should be permitted near crashed cars, nor should matches be struck for light. If there are a number of bystanders, ask one of them to act as fireguard.

Use the lights of undamaged vehicles to light up the incident at night, but beware of parking these vehicles in a position of danger when doing this. Shine lights from the edge of the road if possible.

SINGLE AND MULTIPLE CASUALTIES

> With multiple casualties, or if any casualty is severely injured, sending for help must have a high priority.

If a car or cars have overturned, people are liable to be thrown out. Such casualties may be found at some distance from the vehicles and are usually more severely injured than the ones who remain in the car. These casualties must be sought for, especially at night, covering a wide area of search. The purpose of first-aid is to save lives—and casualties cannot be helped if they are not found. Always try to check how many people were in each vehicle, and make sure that you can account for all of them.

EXTRACTION OF TRAPPED CASUALTIES

Rapid rough extraction of trapped casualties may or may not be good first-aid—usually it is not. The only indication for such a procedure is if immediate danger threatens and the casualty is going to be made worse by leaving him—for example, if there is a fire, if the vehicle may fall over an embankment, or if severe bleeding cannot be stopped without getting the casualty out. Generally there is no necessity for very rapid extraction. First-aid can usually be given without moving the trapped casualty, and this is a preferable procedure. When skilled help arrives—usually the fire brigade—the casualty can often be freed without causing further injury. *Always ask for special help if you know that there are trapped casualties. Mention trapped casualties in your first request for help if you possibly can.*

Any injury to the spine, whether in the neck or in the upper or lower part of the back, can easily be made worse by bad handling. Always enquire about pain in the neck or back before attempting to move such casualties. Enquire also as to whether or not they can move their toes, and if they can, ask them to move their legs. If you are in doubt about moving such casualties, always leave them. Support them in the position of maximum comfort, with padding in natural hollows, until further help arrives. If there are arm injuries, put the arm(s) in a sling or an improvised sling such as the jacket turned up and pinned.

A NOTE ABOUT DEATHS FOLLOWING ROAD TRAFFIC INJURIES

Some interesting facts about deaths from obstructed breathing following road injuries are given in Table 7.4.

In Brisbane a study was made of the casualties resulting from 2,214 traffic accidents. Out of 188 deaths, bleeding, asphyxia (obstructed breathing) or bleeding and asphyxia together were the causes of 54 deaths (28·8 per cent).

TABLE 7.4

OBSTRUCTED BREATHING
and
deaths from road injuries
(an analysis of 300 cases dying within 48 hours)

In 40·3 per cent of cases, obstructed breathing was
the SOLE CAUSE or a CONTRIBUTORY CAUSE
of death.

In 14·3 per cent of cases, obstructed breathing was
the SOLE CAUSE of death
(two-thirds of these people died at the scene of injury*)

In 26·0 per cent of cases, obstructed breathing was
a CONTRIBUTORY FACTOR
(one-third of these people died at the scene of injury*).

* The survival period averaged

10–20 minutes,

LONG ENOUGH TO APPLY LIFE-SAVING FIRST-AID

Therefore,
the fate of *40·3 per cent* of people who *died of road injuries* in this in-
vestigation *could have been affected by good first-aid.*

Table 7.5 is given by kind permission from the Brisbane traffic injury survey report. One conclusion which can be drawn from the figures in this table is that the *fate of 28·8 per cent of the casualties who died* of bleeding, asphyxia or from bleeding and asphyxia together *could have been affected by good first-aid*, had the opportunities been available to do this.

Another interesting set of facts about the times of death of 2,856 casualties following road traffic injuries in Brisbane and Adelaide is given here.

TABLE 7.5

Cause of death	Place of death				TOTAL deaths
	At scene of injury	In ambulance	In hospital		
			less than 2 hours	more than 2 hours	
(1) Bleeding	5	3	6	6	20
(2) Asphyxia*	4	4	4	14	26
(3) Both bleeding and asphyxia	3	2	1	2	8
(4) TOTAL of (1), (2), (3) above, i.e. deaths which may be preventable by good first-aid if applied swiftly	(12)	(9)	(11)	(22)	(54)
(5) Other causes	53	16	14	51	134
(6) ALL CAUSES	65	25	25	73	188
(7) Percentage of deaths which might be preventable by good first-aid	18·5	36·0	44·0	30·2	28·7

* presumably due to obstructed breathing.

In general terms,

about *50 per cent* of the deaths occurred within *1 hour*,

about *80 per cent* of the deaths occurred within *1 day*,

about *90 per cent* of the deaths occurred within *1 week*.

Figure 7.1 shows the percentage of deaths plotted against time.

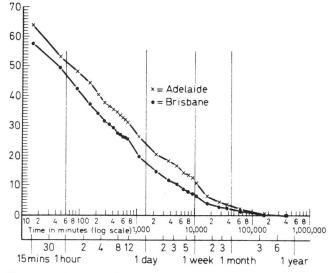

Figure 7.1.—Percentage of all those traffic-accident casualties who eventually died surviving at time shown (Reproduced from Tonge and colleagues by courtesy of the authors and Editor of the 'Lancet')

It may be concluded from this figure and from the previous information in this section that many deaths occur shortly after injury and that a number of these deaths—*probably amounting to at least 25 per cent* could be affected by good first-aid.

233

FIRST-AID for UNCONSCIOUSNESS

Unconsciousness is a great killer in road injuries because it gives rise to obstructed breathing. Obstructed breathing is usually due *either* to a chin-to-chest or other head-forward position allowing the air passages to be blocked, *or* to blood, vomit and secretions blocking the airway whilst casualties are lying on their backs.

> Unconscious casualties are probably the largest single group whose lives can be saved by good first-aid.

The main points of first-aid for unconsciousness are as follows.

(*i*) If the casualty is unconscious and breathing, turn him into the unconscious position (*Figure 7.2*).

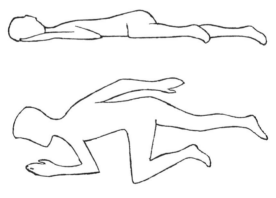

Figure 7.2.—The unconscious position

(*ii*) Clear the mouth of dentures or loose natural teeth and remove any blood, vomit or secretion by blotting out gently with a handkerchief, or, if you have a sucker, by sucking. When you remove dentures, put them in the casualty's pocket or handbag.

(*iii*) Extend the neck fully, getting the head back and the chin up *(Figure 7.3(a))*.

(*iv*) Apply a head-down tip if possible, so that any blood, vomit or secretion can drain out of the mouth and will not drain into the lungs *(Figure 7.3(b))*. *Never leave an unconscious person unattended.*

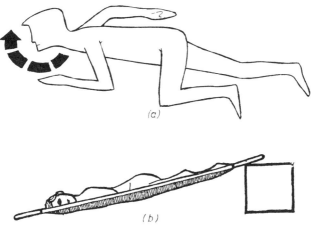

Figure 7.3.—(a) Full head and neck extension in teeth clenched position to keep airway clear. (b) Apply a head-down tip

Any casualty who is unconscious and not breathing should, of course, be given artificial respiration. The mouth-to-nose method is best, but if the nose is blocked, use the mouth-to-mouth method.

Always remove keys or any large hard objects from the pockets of unconscious casualties before loading them on to a stretcher because injury may result in transit from such objects—and unconscious casualties cannot complain of pain.

UNCONSCIOUSNESS AND OTHER INJURIES

Unconscious casualties often have other injuries—especially chest injuries, abdominal injuries and broken limbs. Because the casualty is unconscious, he will not be able to complain of pain or to tell you about these injuries. Therefore, if the correct and appropriate first-aid treatment has to be given, unconscious casualties require very careful examination, after first finding out, if possible, what happened from someone who saw the incident in which the injury was sustained. If the injuries are not discovered, they cannot be treated. Remember that more things are missed by not looking than by not knowing.

BLEEDING

Bleeding must be recognized at once and quickly treated. External bleeding should be dealt with by pressing where the blood comes from, by firm bandaging of dressings and, if other injuries permit, by limb elevation. Internal bleeding can only be effectively treated in hospital; therefore, if internal bleeding is suspected or recognized, that casualty should have a high priority in reaching hospital soon.

SCOOPING UP AND PANIC HANDLING

In the minds of many people who are untrained in first-aid, speed in scooping the casualty off the road surface and loading him into an ambulance is an indication that the job of first-aid was well done. While this may be true in some cases, it is open to question in others—and others are in the majority! Panic handling helps nobody—the casualty suffers increased pain and may have his injuries made worse by such 'treatment'. The first-aider blunts his judgment by allowing himself to be rushed into doing anything.

Beware also of carrying out procedures of little or no real value in an attempt to do something. A cool, calm examination of the situation and of the casualty or casualties will lead to a judgment of what should be done and when, and thus to a correct assessment of the priorities. The correct assessment of injuries is very important, for it is mainly on this that individual priorities are evaluated.

While there is a need not to waste time, there is also a very important need *to spend time in trying to assess both the number and the severity of injuries sustained* by any individual. As we have remarked before, 'more may be missed by not looking than by not knowing'. Experience in many cases shows that

> *more deliberation is indicated at the site of the incident,* and that *the short time spent in getting priorities properly evaluated can save lives.*

When a plan of action is formulated, the arrival of an ambulance should not alter the assessment of what has to be done or when, except to indicate that seriously injured casualties who have been given the necessary first-aid can now be taken to hospital.

SKILLED NEGLECT OF UNIMPORTANT INJURIES

When faced with serious injuries, the need is to carry out the minimum first-aid in order to save the life of the casualty and then to get the casualty to hospital. Correct priorities must be thought out and acted upon. For example, a casualty who is bleeding internally and unconscious from a head injury will require to be taken to hospital without delay, after being treated for unconsciousness. His need is blood replacement for the blood loss which is occurring. This blood replacement and the further management of his head injuries normally can only be carried out in hospital. It is therefore useless to delay his arrival in hospital by splinting a fracture of his little finger and elaborately bandaging a gravel graze of the knee which is not bleeding. Neither of these conditions is life-threatening. The others are.

COMMUNICATION WITH THE HOSPITAL BY PAPER AND PENCIL AND BY RADIO

Not enough use is made of the simple tools of communication in first-aid. Messages which are written down with a time opposite each observation can be of great value to the doctors in hospital, especially in head injury cases. An example is given in *Figure 7.4* of a useful message from a first-aider.

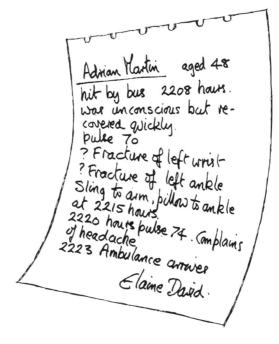

Figure 7.4.—A useful message

Most ambulances are fitted with a radio. Messages can be sent by radio about seriously injured casualties. In this way, the hospital, having had prior notice, is fully prepared to receive the casualty. The radio can also be used to request advice about the management of the casualty. Not enough use is made of this possibility.

CHILDREN AND ELDERLY PEOPLE

Children and elderly people are often involved in road injuries. These two groups tend to withstand the effects of injury and blood loss less well than do fit young or middle-aged adults. Another way of saying this is that injury in a child or an old person will produce greater general effects than a similar injury in a fit adult. Therefore, such casualties should have a higher priority in reaching hospital than adults who have equivalent injuries.

TALK TO CASUALTIES

Talk frequently and reassuringly to conscious casualties. Bewildered casualties may ask the same question many times. Answer the question in a kindly voice each time it is asked. This helps to stop panic and fright, and will gain cooperation from the casualty.

It may be wise in some circumstances to avoid telling seriously injured casualties of the death of another—they will learn soon enough. Temporary lessening of horror by evasion or lying may be justified.

If the casualty is obviously dying, try to comfort him by contact of touch or voice during his final moments. This may help to spare him some suffering in what would otherwise be a lonely and more horrible death.

After you have carried out all the first-aid which is necessary, if there is then a waiting period before ambulance or further help arrives, use this time to talk to the casualties on trivialities rather than discuss the causes and horrors of the incident with bystanders.

PROTECTION OF CASUALTIES

Remember that it is usually more important to have protection *under* a casualty lying on a road or roadside than over him. One blanket or coat is all that will normally be required to cover him, unless the situation is very exposed. A good working rule is two layers under and one on top under normal conditions. It may also be wise to leave some casualties inside cars until ambulances arrive. In this way, casualties can be protected from the weather.

Beware also of bewildered casualties wandering off. They may get into danger on the road or may, especially at night, even get lost. Use bystanders to take charge of such casualties.

A PENULTIMATE PARAGRAPH

During the heat of any incident, always keep calm, be reassuring and direct the work of other people who may be willing to help but do not know what to do unless instructed. Make sure that priorities are carefully observed and that your actions are carried out in the correct order to benefit the casualties. When the incident is finished, think again about what happened, about what you did and why you did it, and ask yourself if there are any lessons to be learned. You will usually find that there are . . . .

Lastly, remember to review your first-aid kit for content and replacement!

PREVENTION

No section about road injuries would be complete without a word on prevention. Most incidents and injuries result from a multiplicity of factors, but the principal cause in most cases is people, not things (*see* page 63).

If a car crash is inevitable, the most important thing which will save the lives of the passengers is that they remain in the vehicle, and do not strike against the steering wheel, windscreen, parcel shelf and so on. To prevent this happening, passengers should be strapped into their seats. The usefulness of seat belts in preventing injuries is now beyond conjecture, doubt or speculation, in spite of much ill-informed opinion to the contrary. The *facts* are that seat belts, *if worn properly*, are the most important life-saving, injury-preventing factor in car design.

HORROR STORIES

> *Experience is the name everyone gives to their mistakes.*
>
> OSCAR WILDE

We give below a few examples of how *not* to do first-aid in the hope that a lesson may be learned from each. The stories are all, unfortunately, true.

OBSTRUCTED BREATHING

Due to bleeding and neglect

Following a traffic injury, a man was found to be unconscious by a radiographer. He was lying on his back, bleeding from the mouth and nose, and blue in colour. She turned him over, and cleared out blood clot and vomit from the mouth and throat with her fingers. He was then breathing easily and became pink.

The casualty was then loaded into an ambulance with an untrained person to 'look after him'. He was dead 7 minutes later when the ambulance arrived at hospital. His mouth and nose became obstructed in a pool of blood, because he was laid on his back.

Due to vomiting, ignorance and bad treatment

A man, who was found lying beneath his bicycle on a road, died 'as a result of misadventure' a coroner decided.

A lady member of a first-aid organization said that she saw the man lying in the road with the cycle on top of him.

'He was trying to speak but could not get his words out', she said. 'He appeared to lapse into unconsciousness and I made him comfortable until the ambulance arrived.'

A pathologist said that death was due to asphyxia caused by vomit blocking the air passages. 'Making him comfortable' probably involved putting his head on a pillow while lying on his back, thus aiding airway obstruction.

BLEEDING

A man was found by a nurse at the scene of a traffic accident holding a pad in front of his right ear. The nurse removed the pad (a mistake), and the casualty was seen to be bleeding from a wound in front of the ear. A small artery was torn. The nurse, finding it difficult to stop the bleeding, directed the casualty to a police car which had arrived at the scene and asked the officer to drive with all speed to the hospital about $4\frac{1}{2}$ miles away. This he did, through heavy traffic at 5·00 p.m. On arrival at hospital the back of the police car was like a blood bath, and the emotional temperature of the scene was operatic.

The casualty sister at the hospital stopped the bleeding at once by pressing where the blood was coming from. The casualty, the so-called nurse or indeed anyone else could have stopped the bleeding by pressing—*and this had in fact been done* by a first-aider before the interference by the nurse. From this skin-deep wound about an inch long, the casualty bled sufficiently to require a transfusion of 4 units of blood. Had he bled more, his life might easily have been lost. When bleeding has been stopped, dressings should not be removed, except in hospital.

The local newspaper next day said 'nurse saves man's life'. Neither the casualty sister nor the doctor agreed!

A FRACTURED SPINE

A motor cyclist crashed into a lorry. He complained of

pain in his back when lying face upwards in the road. In order to let the traffic past, he was picked up under his arms and knees ('jack-knifed'), and was taken to the edge of the road. In the middle of the road he could move his legs and feet, and could feel his toes being touched. This was the last time he could ever do these things. He is now doubly incontinent and will be in a wheelchair for the rest of his life. But the traffic got past without much delay . . . .

FOOLISH 'RESCUERS'

A boy aged 11 years was overcome by leaking gas when playing in a shaft at a building site. Four men, including the boy's father and brother, were overcome one after another as they went down to try to rescue him. The boy and all four men died. Firemen with breathing apparatus arrived just in time to prevent a sixth person from entering the shaft.

ALWAYS READ THE LABEL

A mother gave two spoonsful of what she thought was cough linctus to her child aged 4 years. Six hours later, when the child was unconscious and moribund, she realized that instead of cough linctus she had given the child camphorated oil. Fortunately the child survived. This mother always reads labels now. But what a way to learn!

LOOK FOR CASUALTIES AFTER CAR CRASHES

A man was found in a field adjacent to the site of a car crash which had occurred *2 days previously*. He was alive. Fortunately, he made a good recovery.

CHAPTER 8

FIRST-AID EQUIPMENT AND RESCUE

FIRST-AID EQUIPMENT

INTRODUCTION

Equipment for use in first-aid can be considered in two categories.

(1) basic first-aid kits, and

(2) other first-aid equipment.

BASIC FIRST-AID KITS

Basic first-aid kits should consist of supplies of triangular bandages, large, medium and small wound dressings, safety pins, and paper and pencil. The exact amount of each item should be specified according to the expected emergencies for which the kit provides first-aid materials, and the numbers of first-aiders who will use the kit. A torch should always be available with the kit.

A separate kit should be provided for the home (or definitive) treatment of minor injuries and illnesses because this will be required under quite different circumstances (*see New Essential First Aid* for details of basic first-aid kits).

OTHER FIRST-AID EQUIPMENT

Sucker

The maintenance of a free airway has a very high priority in first-aid procedures and a sucker is a piece of equipment which should be carried in all ambulances and certainly should be available in all first-aid and medical centres.

Suction is much more efficient than wiping and blotting as a means of removing blood, secretions and vomit from the mouth, throat and nose.

Automatic breathing machines in first-aid

The first question to ask is 'why use automatic breathing machines at all?' Artificial respiration by the exhaled air method of mouth-to-nose or mouth-to-mouth breathing offers a better first-aid solution in general to the problem of not breathing than does the use of machines because, except in an non-respirable atmosphere and perhaps in certain cases of poisoning,

—the human equipment necessary to carry out artificial respiration is always available, arrives with the rescuer in working order, and is less liable to breakdown than a machine. There are often spares!

—a machine can run out of oxygen or suffer mechanical breakdown.

—an airtight seal over the nose and/or mouth of the casualty is easily and securely maintained by the rescuer's lips; a machine depends very much on the skill of the operator using the mask provided to get an airtight seal over the mouth and nose. In our experience, only skilled medical personnel are usually capable of this. Extensive initial training and frequent refresher training is required, if first-aiders are to use such machines.

We would therefore suggest that unless the above criteria are anticipated or fulfilled—and this should be judged by an experienced doctor—first-aiders will give better treatment by using exhaled air artificial respiration than by using machines, and should train accordingly. The reader should also refer again to the remarks about the use of oxygen in first-aid on page 21.

In synopsis, therefore, an automatic machine offers advantages over artificial respiration by the exhaled air method *under the following circumstances only:*

—In a non-respirable atmosphere where breathing apparatus should be worn by the rescuer; for example, in the hold of a ship which is filled with poisonous gas or in any oxygen-deficient atmosphere.

—Where artificial respiration by the exhaled air method cannot be carried out; for example, where a rescuer may come into contact with poison on a casualty's lips, mouth or nose.

Once-only handling of stretcher cases using a sheet

Excessive handling usually increases pain and enhances blood loss, thus adversely affecting the general condition of the casualty.

Casualties who have to be transported should be manually handled once only, that is, when being placed on the stretcher or trolley. A carrying sheet should always be on any stretcher on which the casualty is first placed. On arrival at hospital, poles are inserted into the edges of the carrying sheet and spreaders are then applied. The casualty can then be placed without further manual handling on a hospital trolley.

Much needless handling leading to worsening of the casualty's general condition can be avoided by the more widespread use of this simple method.

a note on the maintenance of equipment

All equipment for use in an emergency must be maintained in good condition and must be ready for immediate use. Emergencies occur suddenly and without warning—so it is wise to carry out regular checking of all equipment which may be used. It is also advisable to keep a written record of these checks so that they can be shown to have been carried out in case of equipment failure.

RESCUE

RESCUE AND FIRST-AID

INTRODUCTION

Although the subject of this book is advanced first-aid, we

are including a short section on rescue in the following pages, because rescue is often intimately associated with a need for first-aid, and vice versa. Of necessity, the section on rescue is incomplete. Special circumstances will require special rescue methods. However, we hope that the remarks may be of use to those who have little experience of rescue problems.

In many rescue situations, the first need of the rescuer is to be familiar with the hazards of the situation; the second need is to be trained in first-aid.

For example, in mountain and cave rescue, the rescuers have to be skilled mountaineers or spelaeologists who should, in addition, have a training in first-aid. It is therefore necessary, in selecting people for rescue training, to make sure that they have a sound knowledge of the situations which they will encounter *before* giving them further first-aid training.

First-aid training for rescuers should include a foundation of general first-aid as well as specialized training in first-aid which is related to the particular hazards which may be encountered. It is also advisable to make sure that people selected for training will have a reasonable expectation of being available immediately, should they be required.

In industry, the same principles hold good; the rescuer must have a sound knowledge of the industrial hazards as well as a knowledge of first-aid to be useful—and unless he already knows the hazards, there is no point in including him in a rescue team and giving further rescue or first-aid training.

THE CALCULATED RISK IN RESCUE

Rescue of casualties implies in many, if not most, instances the principle of the calculated risk. The risks to the rescuer must be objectively assessed and acted upon, and the chances of bringing back—or out—a live, treatable casualty have to be weighed. No purpose is served by increasing the number of casualties by would-be rescuers becoming casualties themselves. Nor is there any point in risking lives to bring out the dead. All actions should be based on the degree of risk, weighed with and against the chances of success. This assessment of risk *before* action is essentially the difference between bravery and foolhardiness.

There are several well-documented instances of gas escapes where multiple casualties resulted. In one case the number of the original casualties was doubled by inexperienced 'rescuers' going to 'help' *before* the alarm was sounded; when the properly trained and equipped rescuers came on to the scene they found that their job was twice as large as it should have been. Some of the 'rescuers' in this instance died, while some of the original casualties were rescued and resuscitated.

THE ORGANIZATION OF RESCUE

Pre-planning, attention to detail, adequate equipment, training, enthusiasm, clear-headedness in emergency and good leadership are all ingredients in successful rescue.

As far as possible, plans should be made *in advance* to deal with the kinds of emergency situations which can be foreseen. Such plans can never be complete to the final detail, and good improvisation is always required. However, if a framework exists, the chances are that less on-the-spot improvisation will be required and that a better operation will be carried out because people understand what they should be doing without having to be told.

CHAPTER 9

TEACHING FIRST-AID

In the course of teaching first-aid, and of reviewing the results of current teaching, we have become aware:
—that many problems are tackled by first-aiders without understanding the principle involved (as distinct from the detail),
—that an excess of instruction can serve to cloud an issue which is simple in principle,
—that a few simple rules which are remembered and carried out will tend to be more effective first-aid than half-remembered floundering,
—that attention to breathing and to airway maintenance is less well understood and practised than it needs to be,
—that often the best first-aid will be to do a few simple things effectively and get the casualty comfortably and without delay to hospital, and
—that the principle of the calculated risk should be accepted.

WHAT IS FIRST-AID?

First-aid is the process of carrying out the essential emergency treatment of an injury (or illness) in order to benefit the casualty. The casualty is then sent to hospital (or to a doctor) for further treatment. The treatment of the casualty is *not* completed at the scene of the injury. Treatment is initiated with the understanding that further treatment will be required.

An underlying assumption to normal first-aid training should be that hospital facilities are within reasonable reach, and that help can be summoned.

WHAT FIRST-AID IS NOT

Only aid

The definitive treatment of minor injuries and non-serious conditions could be described as 'only aid'. This will include the definitive treatment of minor injuries at home and in factories. But this is not a part of first-aid as we have defined it; there is no intention of passing the casualty on for further treatment.

In teaching people to do 'only aid', it is necessary to teach both how to apply the correct definitive treatment for the condition, and also how to discriminate between the injuries which should be treated in this way and those injuries which should be given first-aid and passed on for further treatment.

The distinction between first-aid (treatment) and only aid (definitive treatment) is important, and has considerable practical implications.

Rescue

For example, mountain or pot-holing rescue requires that the first-aider must firstly be a mountaineer or a pot-holer and secondly a first-aider. Therefore, the aim should be to train people who are already skilled as mountaineers or pot-holers in the first-aid problems of rescue associated with their particular sport. Highly specialized training will therefore be required.

Medicine at sea or in remote places

This is not a part of first-aid as we have defined it.

Only aid, rescue and medicine at sea or in remote places all have important elements of first-aid—but in each case special additional skills are required.

WHAT GRADE OF FIRST-AID SHOULD BE TAUGHT AND TO WHOM?

LIFE-SAVING AND ELEMENTARY

This should be taught to *all* schoolchildren, so that eventually everyone knows some first-aid. In Norway, the people care sufficiently for their children and about their future as adults in a community that safety, accident prevention and first-aid are taught as a compulsory subject in every school during every term of the child's schooling. These subjects are taught by the ordinary class teachers, with the aid of suitable briefing. As an example, during one term the teacher is required to spend 6 hours of class time teaching you what to do if you find yourself in a burning building; how to escape; how to use a fire extinguisher; how to call the fire brigade; how to give first-aid for heat burns. This sort of teaching in schools on a regular basis to *all* children is surely an example to the world. What subjects are more important or more vital? Omission of this kind of teaching may lose lives—it should therefore be remembered that you cannot teach dead children. Parents may care to ask if these subjects are being taught in the schools to which their children go. If not, why not?

ESSENTIAL (STANDARD ADULT GRADE)

This is the level which any adult who wishes to do first-aid should attain. It is the level which should be aimed at in the ordinary adult textbook of first-aid.

ADVANCED FIRST-AID

People with this level of training are the *élite* of the body of first-aiders. A high standard of knowledge and practice should be required, together with demonstrated aptitude.

This is the level which should be required of ambulance drivers and attendants, of members of over 5 years' duration of the voluntary societies, and of many industrial and rescue first-aiders.

The subsequent remarks apply mainly to adult first-aid teaching.

WHO SHOULD BE TRAINED IN FIRST-AID?

STUDENT NURSES AND MEDICAL STUDENTS

There is a need to teach first-aid to student nurses and to medical students. It is unfortunately true that some state registered nurses and doctors receive as yet no instruction in first-aid as part of their training.

PEOPLE SELECTED FROM THE PUBLIC

Apart from elementary first-aid which should be taught to everyone, people who could be trained in essential and advanced first-aid should be *selected* using some of the following criteria:

intelligence,
personality,
availability, in general and in emergency,
interest and enthusiasm.

In advanced first-aid training, in particular, there is a need to select people and not to take all-comers, regardless of their suitability.

The remarks below relate to essential and advanced first-aid training.

WHO SHOULD TEACH FIRST-AID?

Everyone who teaches first-aid should themselves be interested in the subject and able to convey enthusiasm. The subject must be presented in a stimulating way—a parrot-like repetition of a first-aid book or a reading aloud from the book is guaranteed to send the audience into a self-defensive lack of attention. Good teachers usually enjoy teaching. If the teacher does not enjoy teaching the subject, then it would probably be better for everyone if someone else did the teaching.

School teachers should teach elementary first-aid; doctors and experienced first-aiders should teach essential first-aid and advanced first-aid. The participation by doctors should be relatively more in advanced first-aid training.

It may also be pertinent to ask who should teach the teachers of first-aid, including doctors, and ascertain that adequate instruction is in fact given. The holding of a medical degree does not in our opinion automatically qualify a person to be an instructor.

HOW SHOULD FIRST-AID BE TAUGHT?

FORM SUITABLE TRAINING GROUPS

Much of the existing first-aid training which is carried out is done on a 'cottage industry' basis—in small groups. Modern transport facilities allow larger groups to be formed without too many problems.

In large towns or cities, and even in country areas, the formation of groups is unnecessarily fragmented under rival first-aid organizations. Surely the time has come in this country when *one* national body could form groups and could co-ordinate and standardize first-aid training. Much senseless rivalry still occurs.

(*a*) *Use large groups for lectures and films; small groups for practical instruction.*—For lectures and formal instruction, large groups should be used. It is as easy to give a lecture to 50 or 500 people as to 5. The quality of the lecture will often be better if the lecturer knows that he has to face a large audience, human nature being what it is! Better lecturers can be engaged if a larger audience is obtained. The costs of such a meeting will often be less, as the overheads can be shared among this larger group. It may be quite simple to justify certain things in large groups which could not be done in small groups.

This sort of approach will, of course, require a great deal of re-thinking and re-organizing by those who arrange first-aid training within the first-aid organizations and in industry.

For practical instruction small groups should be used.

The large groups should be instructed by experienced doctors who are interested in first-aid. The small groups should be trained in practical first-aid by experienced first-aiders of advanced level, under the general supervision of a doctor.

(*b*) *Do not mix grades.*—In the formation of groups for training, new entrants should be segregated from people for re-training to the same level. So, also, should trainees to essential level be segregated from those who are learning advanced first-aid.

AIM FOR SIMPLICITY

(*a*) *Cut redundant information.*—Needless complication and unnecessary anatomy and physiology should be omitted. For example, in teaching artificial respiration by the exhaled air method, there is no need for a discourse on 'alveoli and their lining by flattened cells which cover capillaries of the pulmonary circulating system'. All the important concepts can be illustrated to a class by blowing up a balloon and allowing the air to escape. If the neck of the balloon is obstructed or is bent round the fingers the balloon cannot be inflated—hence the need for an unobstructed and straight airway. The lungs are like balloons.

Similarly a knowledge of the chambers of the heart never helped anyone to stop bleeding from a cut.

(*b*) *Teach one effective method.*—Teach one method, not three, when one will do—for example, teach exhaled air artificial respiration and omit Holger–Neilson, Schafer, Sylvester and other methods. Similarly, do not teach what *not* to do. Teach the correct method of doing things—for example, how to stop bleeding by pressing where the blood comes from, by lifting up the injured part higher than the heart and by keeping the injured part still to prevent break up of clot. Omit any mention of pressure points, elastic bandages and tourniquets.

USE THE CALCULATED RISK PRINCIPLE

This principle is that if the correct and beneficial treatment for a certain condition is, in 99 cases out of 100 (or some such number), to do a certain thing, but that to do this in 1 case out of 100 may result in less favourable or unfortunate results, we accept the 1 : 100 risk and act.

The correct treatment of unconsciousness provides a good example. The instructions are that all unconscious persons should, after having the mouth cleared quickly of dentures, loose teeth, blood, vomit or debris, be turned into the unconscious (semi-prone) position, if possible with a slight head-down tip.

There is no doubt that the great majority of unconscious casualties will benefit by this treatment—indeed there is evidence that just over 20 per cent of one sample of 200 road deaths was due to nothing else but blood or vomit blocking the airway. These and many other lives could be saved by the application of the simple rules for the treatment of unconsciousness. There will be a very occasional unconscious casualty, however, who may suffer serious injury by being turned—for example, the casualty with the broken neck.

The dilemma is whether to teach all the possible exceptions—with the result that the first-aider becomes confused or spends a lot of time doing useless checking (which he may or may not do well or be able to do effectively) instead of getting on with vital first-aid measures, *or* whether to take a calculated risk and teach a few simple steps which can be easily remembered, and which should be well carried out, and which in the overwhelming majority of cases will prove to be effective in saving lives. We are indebted to Dr Robert A. Mustard who has stated this principle with great clarity in the excellent book of which he is the author, *The Fundamentals of First Aid.*

STRESS PRIORITIES

The correct order of doing things is poorly appreciated by

many first-aiders—for example, one of us attended a road injury where the casualty was not breathing. There had been no brief examination to find out the condition of the casualty, but a dash to the telephone to summon an ambulance. Full neck extension allowed him to breathe and thus produced a live casualty. In serious cases, skilled neglect of trivial injuries can be life-saving.

Good contemporary first-aid could be described as the art of doing a few things well and in the right order, and then getting the casualty to hospital without wasting time.

OMIT JARGON

Jargon should be eliminated—there is no need to talk of the control of haemorrhage, of syncope and vasovagal reactions or of cyanosis (which many people would not immediately understand) when, equally, we could speak of how to stop bleeding, of fainting and of blueness (which most people would understand at once). It does, however, require some effort on the part of the teacher to eliminate jargon. The reward for jargon elimination is an increase in both the clarity of presentation and in comprehension by the audience.

REFRESHER TRAINING IS REQUIRED

Knowledge does not tend to fossilize—people do. New ideas and methods must be learned and accepted. There is, therefore, a constant need to bring knowledge up to date, and to review existing training.

WHAT TEACHING AIDS CAN BE USED?

(i) *A blackboard* and a set of coloured chalks can often illustrate various points. Half-drawn diagrams which are filled in or completed and labelled as the lecture proceeds will make use of the visual memory of the audience in addition to what they hear.

(ii) *Colour slides* of new and untreated injuries are of very great value in teaching first-aid. Many people have never really seen or looked at injuries. If they have, they have often seen blood and then looked away, and do not recognize what they see unless trained in recognition. Colour slides can be used to teach first-aiders how to look, what to look for, and to interpret what they see. An hour spent looking, with a suitable commentary, at a good series of pictures of wounds, burns and fractures will give more information about the diagnosis and treatment of these conditions than 3 hours of talking. In addition, the pictures will be better remembered by most people.

Colour slides can also be 'home-made' to illustrate situations which can be posed—for example, the unconscious position—or to illustrate points in a talk. Many people nowadays own and operate a camera and could use their own camera to produce slides for lecture purposes.

(iii) *Film strips* can be used in the same way as colour slides.

(iv) *Films* are a very valuable way of teaching *if they are good*. It is wise to view any film *before* showing it to a class!

(v) *Faked casualties.*—Casualties Union have improved casualty faking to a fine art. Their services are available to interested groups. For classes of about 20–40 people, a good exercise is to have a faked casualty or casualties and to have two or three class members come into the room one at a time and individually diagnose and treat the casualty or casualties in front of the group. A discussion is then held about what should be done and about what was or was not done. Much can be learned in this way. If Casualties Union are not available, experienced first-aiders can, with suitable instruction and make-up, often do a very good job of being a casualty.

(vi) *Television.*—The potentialities of television as a mass instruction medium are under-exploited to the extent that most educational programmes are relegated to the nonpeak-viewing hours. This is a comment on the social phenomena of our times, and the relative values of education and entertainment.

(vii) *Competitions.*—We have some doubt about whether this subject should appear under the heading of teaching aids. There is indeed some evidence from first-aid competitions that a curious world of make-believe exists which bears but a fragmentary resemblance to reality. Team theatrical performances disguised as first-aid competitions contribute to this fairyland phenomenon. Should doctors encourage this?

WHAT ABOUT PREVENTION?

First-aid is always a poor second to the prevention of injuries. Not nearly enough is made of the opportunities which arise naturally in the teaching of first-aid to drive home the lessons of prevention. First-aiders and doctors have unique opportunities to foster a preventive approach to injuries, incidents and damage which arises. Most of these so-called accidents are not accidental and are easily preventable. Such injuries are the inevitable end-result of faulty actions, unsafe conditions and a fatalistic attitude towards prevention which, if applied today in the field of infectious diseases, would cause enormous public outcry. Here is an educational and preventive opportunity which should be seized by all concerned.

APPENDICES

1. AIRWAYS AND TUBES IN FIRST-AID

INTRODUCTION

In general, we do not recommend the use of airways and tubes in first-aid unless *expert practical training* is given in their use, and *unless those trained are also made aware of the dangers of improper use*. For these reasons, we have put this discussion as an appendix. Without expertly supervised practical training, airways and tubes can be *misused*, with harmful results.

The following remarks are therefore intended as a supplement to such practical training, and unless such training has been given, airways and tubes should not, in our opinion, be used. While there is unequivocal evidence that apparatus, properly used, can facilitate ventilation, there is also evidence of abuse of apparatus, with resultant hazards.

THE GUEDEL AIRWAY

The Guedel airway (*Figure A.1*) is inserted into the mouth and is then rotated and placed over the top of the tongue,

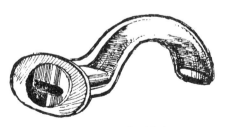

Figure A.1.—A Guedel airway

259

coming to rest with the flap end of the airway inside the lips and outside the teeth (*Figure A.2*).

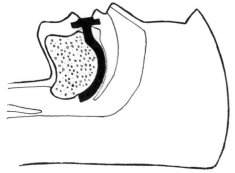

Figure A.2.—Guedel airway in use

Dentures should be removed prior to the insertion of the airway. The flap end of the airway then rests inside the lips and outside the jaws.

The airway will stop the tongue from falling back in an unconscious casualty. Several sizes of airway should be carried.

AIRWAYS FOR GIVING ARTIFICIAL RESPIRATION

These airways are of use to remove aesthetic objections to giving mouth-to-mouth artificial respiration. They offer no significant advantage, except the aesthetic one, over the no-apparatus methods.

AIR-BAG-TYPE RESUSCITATORS

Air-bag-type resuscitators ('Ambu bag', 'air-viva' and so on) use an anaesthetic-type face mask over the mouth and nose. Air is blown by squeezing the bag. Oxygen can be introduced into the face mask through a side tube.

The problems associated with this apparatus are those of the juggler—how to maintain an airtight seal on the face mask by pressing *down*, while at the same time supporting the lower jaw by pulling *upwards*, to prevent the tongue falling back, and also maintaining full neck extension, using one hand only; the other hand is used to squeeze the bag and blow air in.

If people can be adequately trained to perform this difficult feat and they are in possession of the requisite apparatus, then they can give artificial respiration by this method.

The under-trained or unskilled person using the air-bag type of resuscitator usually begins by pushing the face mask firmly downwards, thus flexing the neck and allowing the jaw to sag. This may easily aggravate or produce airway obstruction.

It is, however, our experience that much better ventilation is performed by most people when doing artificial respiration by the mouth-to-nose or mouth-to-mouth methods. All the necessary apparatus for these methods arrives with the rescuer in full working order.

2. USEFUL HANDOUTS AND POSTERS

POCKET FIRST AID*

This is a small glazed pocket-sized card which teaches in line with *New Essential First Aid* and *New Advanced First-aid*. It is in six main sections: priorities; life-saving first-aid; first-aid to prevent worsening; poisoning by mouth; clothing on fire; road crashes.

INSTANT FIRST AID*

This is a poster which teaches in line with *New Essential First Aid* and *New Advanced First-aid* and which is laid out similarly to *Pocket First Aid*. The two are complementary.

SURVIVAL AT SEA*

This small glazed pocket-sized card is set out in five sections: priorities of survival; wet-cold chilling (hypothermia); raft capsize; rescue and life-saving first-aid. The centre-page spread gives detailed information about how to survive under three main headings: abandoning ship to boarding the life-raft (lifeboat); boarding the life-raft and the first 24 hours; after the first 24 hours.

* Available from Lyndhurst Printing Company, Hardley, Hythe, Southampton (telephone no.: Hythe (0703) 846334).

3. USEFUL BOOKS

New Essential First Aid (Pan, London, 1984)
This is a companion volume to *New Advanced First-aid* by the same authors.

Principles for First Aid to the Injured, by H. Proctor and P. S. London (Butterworths, London, 1977)
A useful and interesting book which is written by experts from the Birmingham Accident Hospital.

INDEX

INDEX

INDEX

INDEX

INDEX